ANATOMY OF SPORTS INJURIES

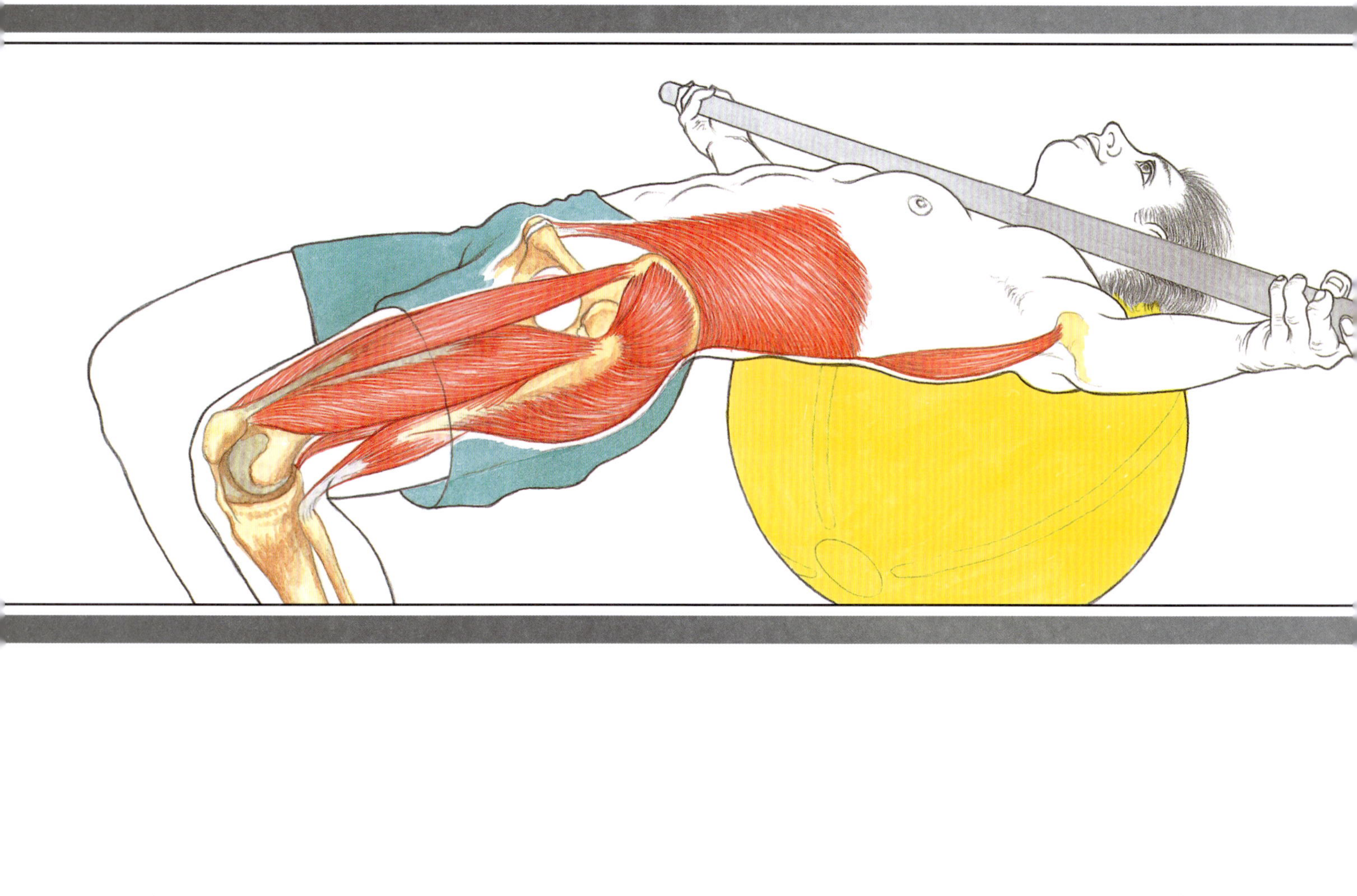

ANATOMY OF SPORTS INJURIES

FOR FITNESS AND REHABILITATION

LEIGH BRANDON

IMM lifestyle books™
Read. Learn. Do What You Love.

Text, illustrations, and photographs by IMM Lifestyle Books, an imprint of Fox Chapel Publishing, 903 Square Street, Mount Joy, PA 17552. *www.foxchapelpublishing.com*.

First Published, Copyright © 2011 IMM Lifestyle Books, an imprint of Fox Chapel Publishing.

Publisher: Guy Hobbs
Senior Editor: Marilyn Inglis
Designer: Peter Crump
Colour illustrations: James Berrangé
Black and white illustrations: Stephen Dew
Production: Marion Storz

ISBN 978-1-5048-0181-2

Printed in China
Second Printing

MIX
Paper | Supporting responsible forestry
FSC® C147414

CONTENTS

PART 1
OVERVIEW OF ANATOMY AND INJURIES

PART 2
COMMON SPORTS INJURIES

PART 3
REHABILITATION

MOBILIZATIONS AND STRETCHES

EXERCISES

PART 1 – OVERVIEW OF ANATOMY AND INJURIES

HOW TO USE THIS BOOK

Anatomy of Sports Injuries for Fitness and Rehabilitation is a visual and textual analysis of common sports injuries and rehabilitation of those injuries through effective exercises. It is also a guide to how to do the exercises properly and when to seek professional help to overcome your sports injury.

The book has three distinct parts: the first is a basic introduction to anatomical definitions, terminology and an overview of sports injuries. It also includes guidelines on injury prevention, acute care and first aid, manual therapy, long-term rehabilitation and lifestyle considerations.

Part Two is divided into 13 sections, each covering a region of the body and highlighting some of the most common injuries for that region. Each section defines individual injuries and their potential causes, treatment plans and statistics. Up to three mobilizations, stretches and/or exercises that may be used to help rehabilitate the injury are suggested as part of the corrective exercise programme following the acute phase of the injury.

Note that an injury can have many different causes and should be assessed by a trained professional to find the underlying causes. Any muscle imbalances should be highlighted at this stage and proper corrective stretching and strengthening should be given based on this information. Without a thorough assessment, the likelihood of full rehabilitation is greatly reduced, therefore, the stretches and exercises recommended may not be applicable to all.

Disclaimer: Many of the exercises have a degree of risk of injury if done without adequate instruction and supervision. We recommend that you have a thorough assessment with a CHEK Practitioner, physiotherapist, osteopath or chiropractor before undertaking any of the exercises, and that you seek qualified instruction if you are a complete beginner. This book does not constitute medical advice and the author and publisher cannot be held liable for any loss, injury or inconvenience sustained by anyone using this book or the information contained in it.

Part Three is an exercise section – a 'how-to' guide to doing the exercises as well as a visual and technical exercise analysis describing which muscles are being used. The start and finish positions are usually depicted and training tips may be included.

The adult human body has more than 600 muscles and 206 bones; in this book, emphasis is placed on about 92 muscles involved in movement and stabilization. Many of the smaller muscles, as well the deep, small muscles of the spine and muscles of the hands and feet are not given specific attention.

This book is designed to help you improve your understanding of sports injuries and to overcome them and get back to performing at your best without the worry of further or future injury. Before starting a rehabilitation programme, the reader is advised to fully understand what phase of recovery they are in and introduce the right treatments and exercises at the right time (explained in Part One). For instance, if stretches and exercises are used in the acute phase, this may further damage tissues and make the injury worse. Therefore, it is advised that you work through the book in the order it was written. In Part One, you will understand the anatomical definitions and terminology used in the book as well as a basic understanding of injuries and rehabilitation strategies. In Part Two you will learn about your injury, while in Part Three you will learn how to perform the exercises and stretches.

Ultimately, the injured tissues need to be conditioned to take the rigours of your sport in all planes of motion. This is known as end-stage rehabilitation. While it is beyond the scope of this book to teach you end-stage rehab, the reader is advised to receive professional advice on strength and conditioning or read *Anatomy of Strength and Fitness Training for Speed and Sport* by Leigh Brandon.

How to perform this exercise

Exercise name

How to start or finish the exercise, as shown in the small artwork

Labels for the major muscles being used during the exercise

TOUCH TOE DRILL

Basic description:

- Inhale, then gently draw your navel in towards your spine.
- Keeping your standing foot fully on the ground, bend the same knee, then reach with the other foot as far forwards as possible.
- Tap the moving foot on the floor at the furthest point you can reach without placing any body weight on the moving foot.
- Repeat at 45° forwards, sideways, 45° backwards, and straight back.
- Repeat on the other side.

STARTING POSITION
- Stand with a dowel across your upper back, then lift one leg.

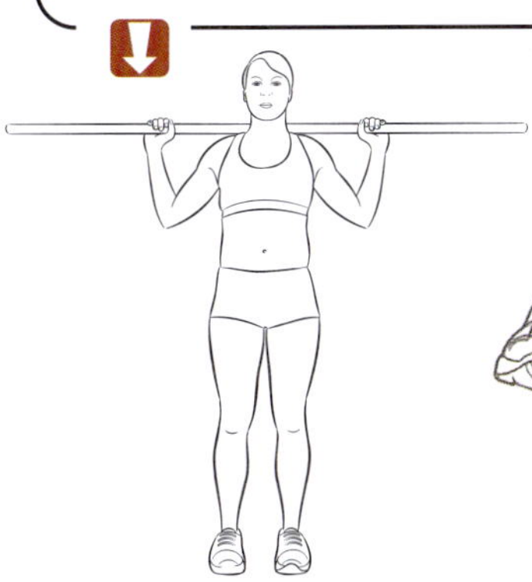

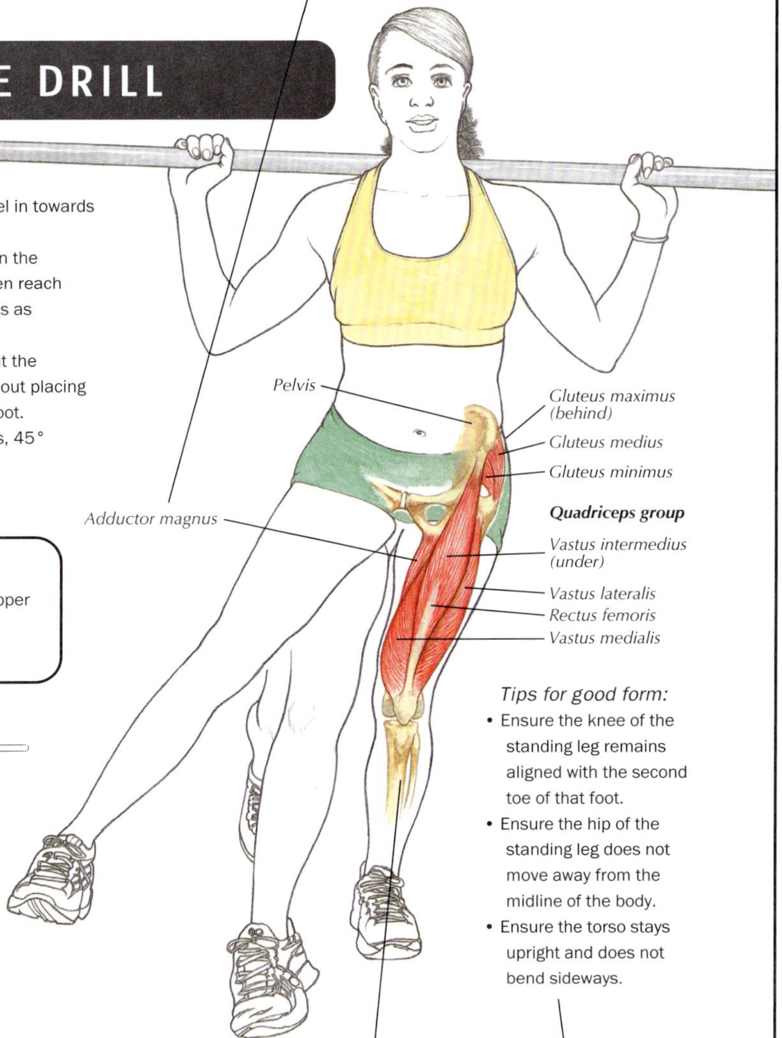

Tips for good form:
- Ensure the knee of the standing leg remains aligned with the second toe of that foot.
- Ensure the hip of the standing leg does not move away from the midline of the body.
- Ensure the torso stays upright and does not bend sideways.

ANALYSIS OF MOVEMENTre-vis	JOINTS	JOINT MOVEMENT	MOBILIZING MUSCLES
Joint 1	Hip	Up: extension Down: flexion	Gluteus maximus, gluteus medius (posterior fibres), biceps femoris, semitendinosus, semimembranosus, adductor magnus (posterior fibres)
Joint 2	Knee	Up: extension Down: flexion	Rectus femoris, vastus medialis, vastus intermedius, vastus lateralis
Joint 3	Ankle	Up: plantarflexion Down: dorsiflexion	Gastrocnemius, soleus, tibialis posterior, peroneus longus and b

7 *REHABILITATION*

Technical aspects, describing the joints, joint movement and mobilizing muscles

Illustration depicting the major muscles used in the exercise

Essential training guidelines

ANATOMICAL DEFINITIONS AND TERMINOLOGY

Anatomy has its own language and although technical, it is quite logical, originating from Latin and Greek root words that make it easier to learn and understand the names of muscles, bones and other anatomy parts.

Whether you are an athlete, a student, a physio-therapist, a strength and conditioning coach or a CHEK practitioner, using the correct words and terminology enables you to interact with other professionals and professional materials.

Like most medical terms, anatomical terms are made up of small word parts, known as combining forms that fit together to make the full term. These 'combining forms' comprise roots, prefixes and suffixes. Knowing the different word parts allows you to unravel the word. Most anatomical terms only contain two parts: either a prefix and root or a root and suffix.

For example, take the terms 'subscapular' and 'suprascapular'; the root is 'scapula', more commonly known as the shoulder blade. 'Supra' means 'above', hence 'suprascapula' means something above the shoulder blade. On the other hand, 'sub' means 'below', indicating in this instance something below the shoulder blade.

Common prefixes, suffixes and roots of anatomical terms

Word root	Meaning	Example	Definition
abdomin	pertaining to the abdomen	abdominal muscle	major muscle group of the abdominal region
acro	extremity	acromion	protruding feature on the scapula bone
articul	pertaining to the joint	articular surface	joint surface
brachi	pertaining to the arm	brachialis	arm muscle
cerv	pertaining to the neck	cervical vertebrae	the neck region of the spine
crani	skull	cranium	bones forming the skull
glute	buttock	gluteus maximus	buttock muscle
lig	to tie, to bind	ligament	joins bone to bone
pector	chest region	pectoralis major	chest muscle
Word parts used as prefixes			
ab-	away from, from, off	abduction	movement away from the midline
ad-	increase, adherence, toward	adduction	movement towards the midline
ante-, antero-	before, in front	anterior	front aspect of the body
bi-	two, double	biceps brachii	two-headed arm muscle
circum-	around	circumduction	circular movement of a limb
cleido-	the clavicle	sternocleiomastoid	muscle, inserts into clavicle
con-	with, together	concentric contraction	contraction in which muscle attachments move together

Word parts used as prefixes (continued)

Word root	Meaning	Example	Definition
costo-	rib	costal cartilage	rib cartilage
cune-	wedge	cuneiform	wedge-shaped foot bone
de-	down from	depression	downward movement of the shoulder blades
dors-	back	dorsiflexion	movement of the top side of the foot towards the shin
ec-	away from	eccentric contractions	contraction in which muscle attachments move apart
epi-	upon	epicondyle	feature of a bone, located above a condyle
fasci-	band	tensor fasciae latae	small band-like muscle of the hip
flex-	bend	flexion	movement closing the angle of a joint
infra-	below, beneath	infraspinatus	muscle situated below the spine of the scapula
meta-	after, behind	metatarsals	bones of the foot, distal to the tarsals
post-	after, behind	posterior	rear aspect of the body
pron-	bent forward	prone position	lying face down
proximo-	nearest	proximal	nearest the root of a limb
quadr-	four	quadriceps	four-part muscle group on the anterior thigh
re-	back, again	retraction	pulling of the shoulder blades towards the midline
serrat-	saw	serratus anterior	muscle with a saw-like edge
sub-	beneath, inferior	subscapularis	muscle beneath the scapula
super, supra-	over, above, excessive	supraspinatus	muscle above the spine of the scapula
		superior	toward the head
thoraco-	the chest, thorax	thoracic vertebrae	in the region of the thorax
trans-	across	transverse abdominus	muscle crossing the abdomen
tri-	three	triceps brachii	three-headed muscle of the upper arm
tuber-	swelling	tubercle	small rounded projection on a bone
Word parts used as suffixes			
-al, ac	pertaining to	iliac crest	pertaining to the ilium
-cep	head	biceps brachii	two-headed arm muscle
-ic	pertaining to	thoracic vertebrae	pertaining to the thorax
-oid	like, in the shape of	rhomboid	upper back muscle, in the shape of a rhomboid
-phragm	partition	diaphragm	muscle separating the thorax and abdomen

SYSTEMS OF THE BODY

The human body can be viewed as an integration of approximately 12 distinct systems that continuously interact to control a multitude of complex functions. These systems are a co-ordinated assembly of organs, each with specific capabilities, whose tissue structures suit a similar purpose and function.

This book illustrates and analyzes the systems that control movement and posture, namely the muscular and skeletal systems, often referred to jointly as the musculoskeletal system.

The other systems are the cardiovascular, lymphatic, nervous, endocrine, integumentary, respiratory, digestive, urinary, immune and reproductive systems.

The muscular system

The muscular system facilitates movement, maintenance of posture and the production of heat and energy. It is made up of three types of muscle tissue: cardiac, smooth and striated.

Cardiac muscle forms the walls in the heart, while smooth muscle tissue is found in the walls of internal organs such as the stomach and blood vessels. Both are activated involuntarily via the autonomic nervous system and hormonal action.

Striated muscle makes up the bulk of the muscles as we commonly know them. The skeletal system includes the tendons that attach muscle to bone, as well as the connective tissue that surrounds the muscle tissue, which is called fascia.

A human male weighing 70 kg (154 lbs) has approximately 25–35 kg (55–77 lbs) of skeletal tissue.

Muscle attachments

Muscles attach to bone via tendons. The attachment points are referred to as the origin and the insertion.

The origin point is the point of attachment that is proximal (closest to the root of a limb) or closest to the midline, or centre of the body. It is usually the least moveable point, acting as the anchor in muscle contraction.

The insertion point is the point of attachment that is distal (the furthest from the root of a limb) or furthest from the midline or centre of the body. The insertion point is usually the most moveable part, and can be drawn towards the origin point.

Knowing the origin and insertion points of a muscle, which joint or joints the muscle crosses and what movement is caused at that joint or joints is a key element of exercise analysis.

There are typical features on all bones that act as convenient attachment points for the muscles. A description of typical bone features is given in the table on page 11.

Muscle attachments

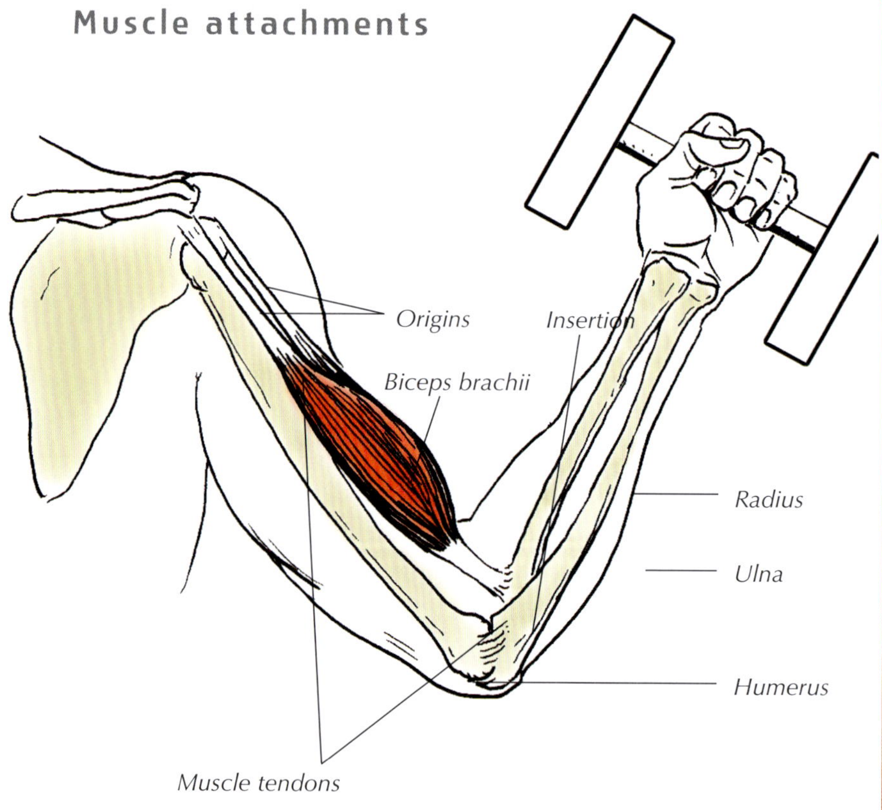

Typical features on a bone

Feature	Description	Examples
Condyle	Large, rounded projection at a joint that usually articulates with another bone	Medial and lateral condyle of the femur Lateral condyle of the tibia
Epicondyle	Projection located above the condyle	Medial or lateral epicondyle of the humerus
Facet	Small, flat joint surfaces	Facet joints of the vertebrae
Head	Significant, rounded projection at the proximal end of a bone, usually forming a joint	Head of the humerus
Crest	Ridge-like, narrow projection	Iliac crest of the pelvis
Line, Linea	Lesser significant ridge, running along a bone	Linea aspera of the femur
Process	Any significant projection	Coracoid and acromion process of the scapula Olecranon process of the ulna at the elbow joint
Spine, Spinous process	Significant, slender projection away from the surface of the bone	Spinous processes of the vertebrae Spine of the scapula
Suture	Joint line between two bones forming a fixed or semi-fixed joint	Sutures that join the bones of the skull
Trochanter	Very large projection	Greater trochanter of the femur
Tubercle	Small, rounded projection	Greater tubercles of the humerus
Tuberosity	Large, rounded or roughened projection	Ischial tuberosities on the pelvis
Foramen	Rounded hole or opening in a bone	The vertebral foramen running down the length of the spine, in which the spinal cord is housed
Fossa	Hollow, shallow or flattened surface on a bone	Supraspinous and infraspinous fossa on the scapula

The word 'skeleton' originates from a Greek word meaning 'dried-up'. Infants are born with about 350 bones, many of which fuse as they grow, forming single bones, resulting in the 206 bones found in an adult.

The muscular system

Anterior view

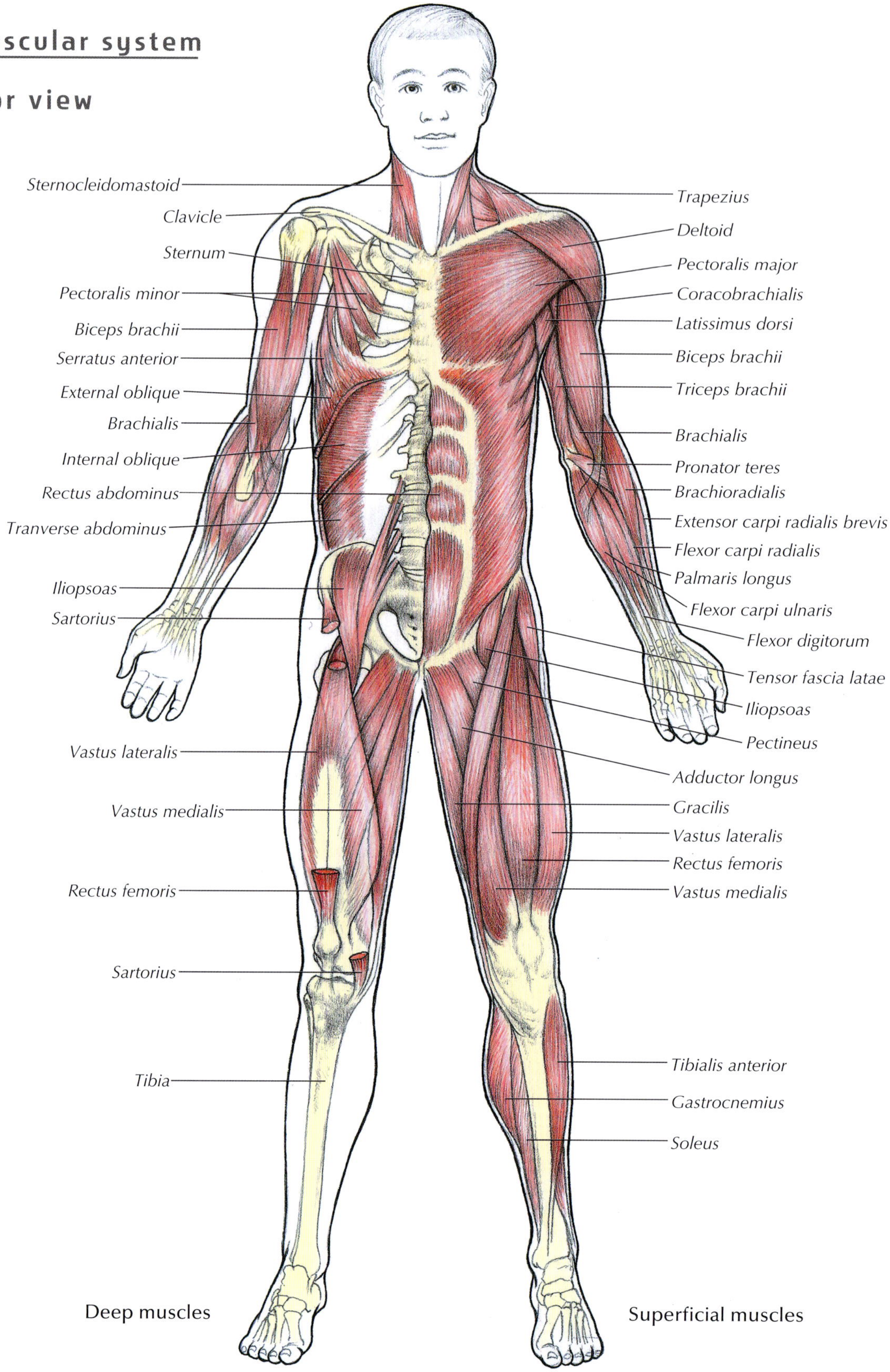

The muscular system

Posterior view

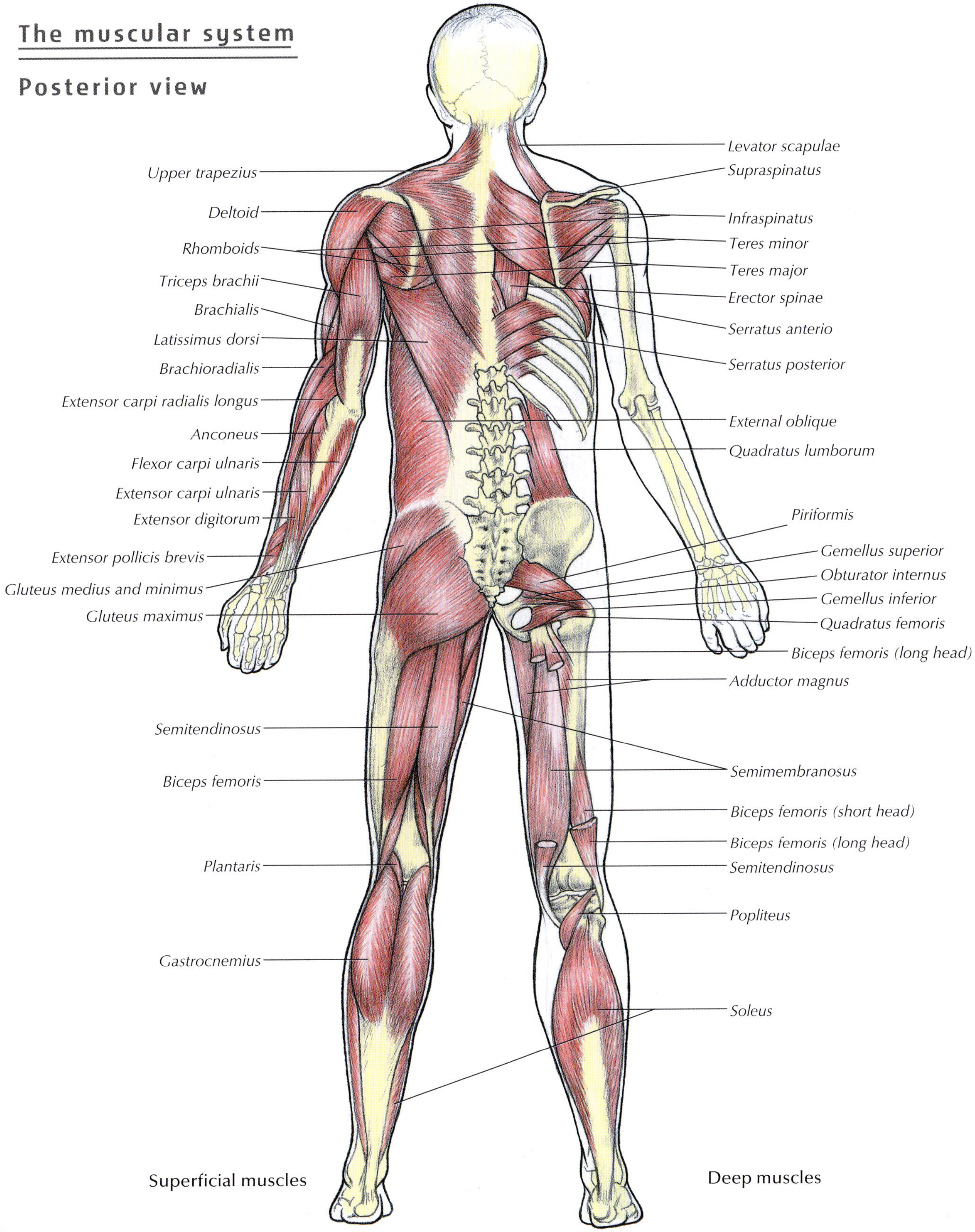

The skeletal system

This consists of bones, ligaments (which join bone to bone) and joints. Joints are referred to as articulations and are sometimes classified as a separate system, the articular system.

Apart from facilitating movement, the primary functions of the skeletal system include supporting the muscles, protecting the soft tissues and internal organs, the storage of surplus minerals and the formation of red blood cells in the bone marrow of the long bones.

Integrated systems

The body's systems are completely and intricately interdependent. For movement to take place, for example, the respiratory system brings in oxygen and the digestive system breaks down our food into essential nutrients. The cardiovascular system then carries the oxygen and nutrients to the working muscles via the blood to facilitate the energy reactions that result in physical work being done.

The lymphatic and circulatory systems help to carry away the waste products of these energy reactions, which are later converted and/or excreted by the digestive and urinary systems. The nervous system interacts with the muscles to facilitate the contraction and relaxation of the muscle tissue. The articular system of joints allows the levers of the body to move.

The skeletal system

Anterior view

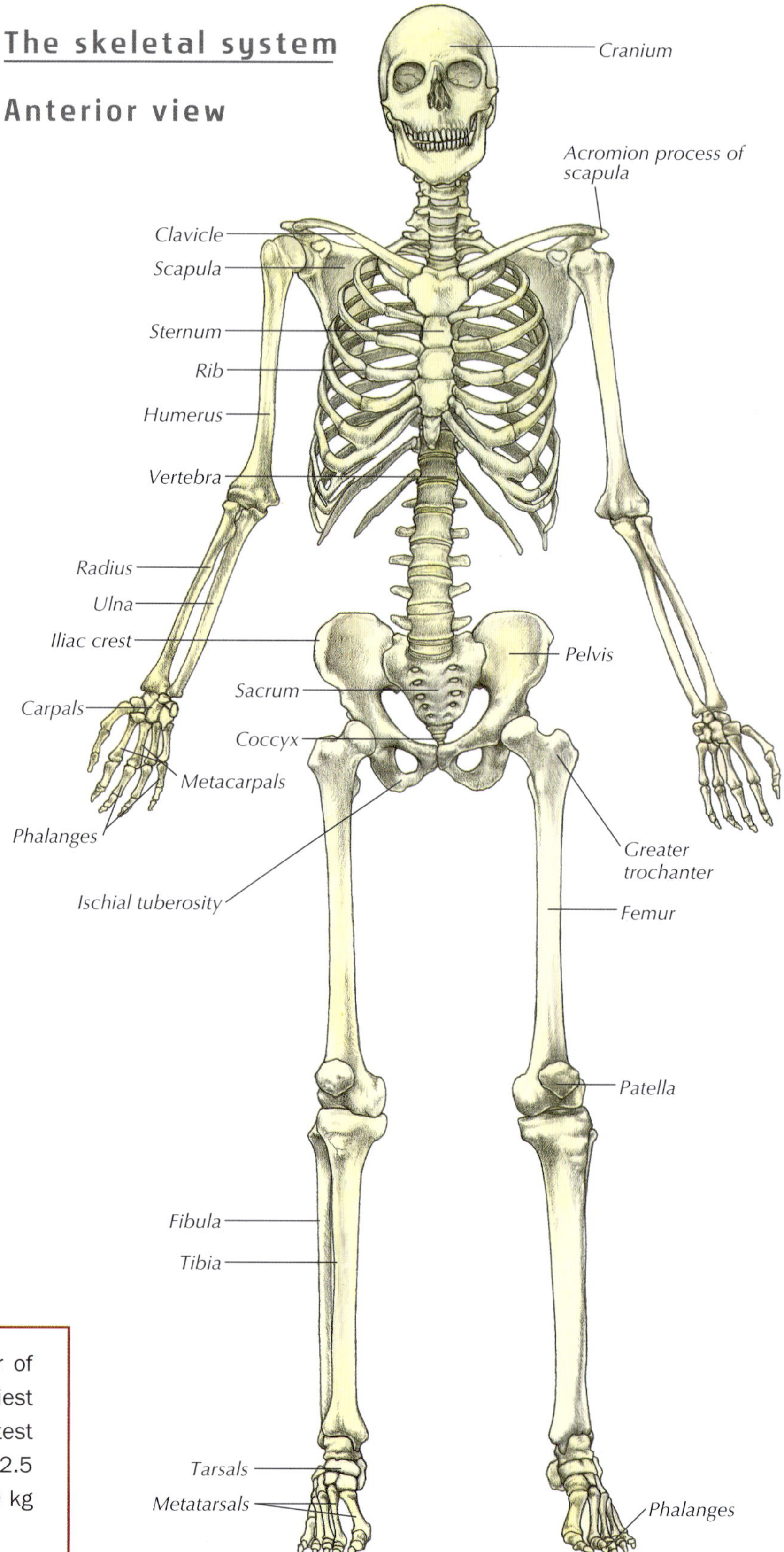

The femur (thigh bone) is about one-quarter of a person's height. It is also the largest, heaviest and strongest bone in the body. The shortest bone, the stirrup bone in the ear is only about 2.5 mm long. An adult's skeleton weighs about 9 kg (20 lb)

BODY PLANES AND REGIONS

When learning anatomy and analyzing movement, we refer to a standard reference position of the human body, known as the anatomical position (see illustrations below). All movements and locations of anatomical structures are named as if the person were standing in this position.

Regional anatomy

This book is a technical labelling guide to the different superficial parts of the body. In anatomical language, common names such as 'head' are replaced with anatomical terms derived from Latin, such as 'cranial' or 'cranium'.

Within the different body regions there are sub-regions. For example, within the cranial region are the frontal, occipital, parietal and temporal sub-regions.

Anatomical planes

The body can be divided into three imaginary planes of reference, each perpendicular to the other.

The sagittal plane passes through the body from front to back, dividing it into a right half and a left half. The midline of the body is called the median. If the body is divided in the sagittal plane, directly through its median, this is known as the median sagittal plane. The coronal (frontal) plane passes through the body from top to bottom, dividing it into front and back sections.

The transverse (horizontal) plane passes through the middle of the body at right angles, dividing it into a top and a bottom section.

An anatomical cross-section of the internal structures of the body can be viewed in any one of these planes, which are also described as 'planes of motion', as the joint movements are defined in relation to one of the three planes. Understanding into which plane an anatomical cross-section is divided will help you know what you are looking at and from which viewpoint.

Anatomical position

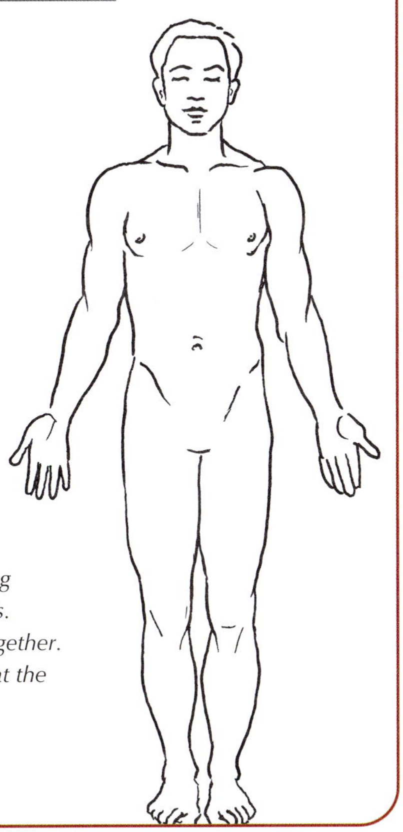

- *The body is in a standing position, facing forwards.*
- *The legs and feet are together.*
- *The arms hang loosely at the sides with palms facing forwards.*

Anatomical planes

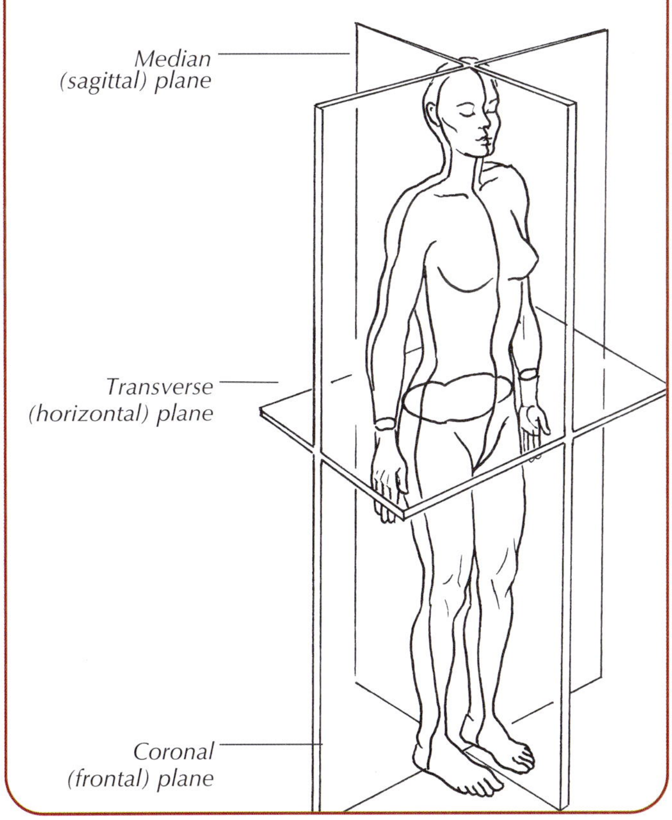

ANATOMICAL TERMS OF POSITION

There are standard anatomical terms that describe the position or direction of one structure of the body and its relationship to other structures or parts of the body.

The human body is a complex, three-dimensional structure. Knowing the proper anatomical terms of position and direction will help you to compare one point on the body with another and understand where it is situated in relation to the other anatomical features. These terms are standard, regardless of whether the person is standing, seated or lying down, and are named as if the person was standing in the anatomical position (see page 12). The terms of direction should not be confused with the labelling of joint movements (see pages 17–20).

Anatomical terms of position and direction

Position	Definition	Example of usage
Anterior	Towards the front, pertaining to the front	The pectoral muscles are found on the anterior aspect of the body
Posterior	Towards the back, pertaining to the back	The calf muscles are situated on the posterior surface of the lower leg
Superior	Above another structure, towards the head	The knee is superior to the ankle
Inferior	Below another structure, towards the feet	The hip is inferior to the shoulder
Lateral	Away from the midline, on or towards the outside	The radial bone is lateral to the ulna
Medial	Towards the midline, pertaining to the middle or centre	The tibial bone is medial to the fibula
Proximal	Closest to the trunk or root of a limb; sometimes used to refer to the origin of a muscle	The shoulder joint is proximal to the elbow
Distal	Situated away from the midline or centre of the body, or root of a limb; sometimes used to refer to a point away from the origin of a muscle	The knee joint is distal to the hip
Superficial	Closer to the surface of the body, more towards the surface of the body than another structure	The rectus abdominus is the most superficial muscle of the abdominal wall
Deep	Further from the surface, relatively deeper into the body than another structure	The transverse abdominus is the deepest muscle of the abdominal wall
Prone	Lying face down	A prone cobra exercise is performed from a lying start position
Supine	Lying on the back, face upwards	A bench press exercise is performed from a supine position

JOINT MOVEMENTS

Knowing and understanding movement (which joint is moving and how it moves) is essential in order to analyze a complex exercise. This book has done the job of joint identification for you, and understanding this section will help improve your exercise analysis.

Types of joints

Some joints are fixed or semi-fixed, allowing little or no movement. For instance, the bones of the skull join together in structures known as sutures to form fixed joints. But where the spine joins the pelvis, the sacroiliac ('sacro' from sacrum and 'iliac' pertaining to the pelvic crest) joint is semi-fixed and allows minimal movement.

A third category, called synovial joints, are free-moving and move in different ways determined by their particular shape, size and structure.

Synovial joints are the most common joints in the body. They are categorized by a joint capsule that surrounds the articulation, the inner membrane of which secretes a lubricating synovial fluid, stimulated by movement. Typical synovial joints include the shoulder, knee, hip, ankle, joints of the feet and hands, and the vertebral joints.

Joint action

When performing an activity such as lifting weights or running, the combination of nerve stimulation and muscular contraction facilitates the movement that occurs at the synovial joints. When doing a deadlift, for example (page 127), the body weight rises away from the floor, because the angle of the ankle, knee and hip joints increases due to the muscles acting across the joints, contracting and causing the joints to extend.

Joint movement pointers

Most joint movements have common names that apply to most major joints, but there are some movements that occur at only one specific joint.

The common joint movements occur in similar anatomical planes of motion. For example, shoulder, hip and knee flexion all occur in the sagittal plane (see page 15). This makes it logical and easier to learn about joint movements and movement analysis. In the table below, common movements are listed first, followed by specific movements that only occur at one specific joint.

Strictly speaking, it is incorrect to name only the movement and a limb or body part. For example, 'leg extension' does not clarify whether this happens at the knee, hip or ankle. Get into the habit of always pairing the movement with the joint that is moved. For example, elbow flexion, hip extension, spinal rotation and scapular elevation. (Possibly the only exception to this is when referring to trunk movements, when all the joints of the spine combine to create movement of the whole body part).

Movements generally occur in pairs. For every movement, there must be a return movement to the starting position. Typical pairs are flexion and extension, abduction and adduction, internal rotation and external rotation, protraction and retraction, elevation and depression.

Remember, all movements are named as if the person was standing in the anatomical position (see page 12). So 'elbow flexion' is the same regardless of whether you are standing, seated or lying (supine).

Major joint movements

General movements	Plane	Description
Abduction	Coronal	Movement away from the midline
Adduction	Coronal	Movement towards the midline
Flexion	Sagittal	Decreasing the angle between two structures
Extension	Sagittal	Increasing the angle between two structures
Medial rotation (internal rotation)	Transverse	Turning around the vertical axis of a bone towards the midline

Lateral rotation (external rotation)	Transverse	Turning around the vertical axis of a bone away from the midline
Circumduction	All planes	Complete circular movement at shoulder or hip joints
Specific movements		
1. Ankle movements		
Plantarflexion	Sagittal	Moving the toes downwards
Dorsiflexion	Sagittal	Moving the foot towards the shin
2. Forearm movements (the radioulnar joint)		
Pronation	Transverse	Rotating the hand and wrist medially from the elbow
Supination	Transverse	Rotating the hand and wrist laterally from the elbow
3. Scapula movements		
Depression	Coronal	Movement of the scapulae inferiorly, e.g. squeezing the scapulae downwards
Elevation	Coronal	Movement of the scapulae superiorly, e.g. hunching the scapulae upwards
Abduction (protraction)	Transverse	Movement of the scapulae away from the spine
Adduction (retraction)	Transverse	Movement of the scapulae towards the spine
Downward rotation	Coronal	Scapulae rotates downwards, in the return from upward rotation
Upward rotation	Coronal	Scapulae rotate upwards.The inferior angle of the scapula moves upwards and laterally
4. Shoulder movements		
Horizontal abduction/extension	Transverse	Movement of the humerus across the body away from the midline
Horizontal adduction/flexion	Transverse	Movement of the humerus across the body towards the midline
5. Spine/trunk movements		
Lateral flexion	Coronal	Movement of the trunk away from the midline
	Coronal	Return of the trunk towards the midline in the coronal plane
6. Wrist movements		
Ulnar deviation	Coronal	Movement of the hand towards the midline from the anatomical position
Radial deviation	Coronal	Movement of the hand away from the midline from the anatomical position

Joint movements

The knee joint is the largest, the hip joint is the strongest, and the shoulder is potentially the most unstable joint in the body.

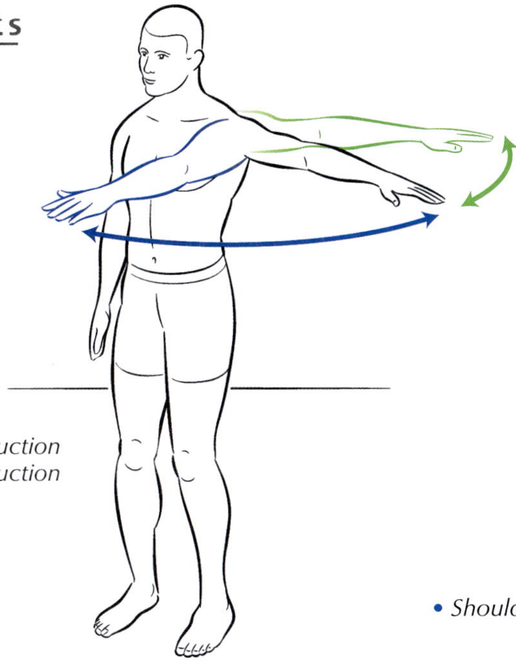

- *Shoulder horizontal adduction*
- *Shoulder horizontal abduction*

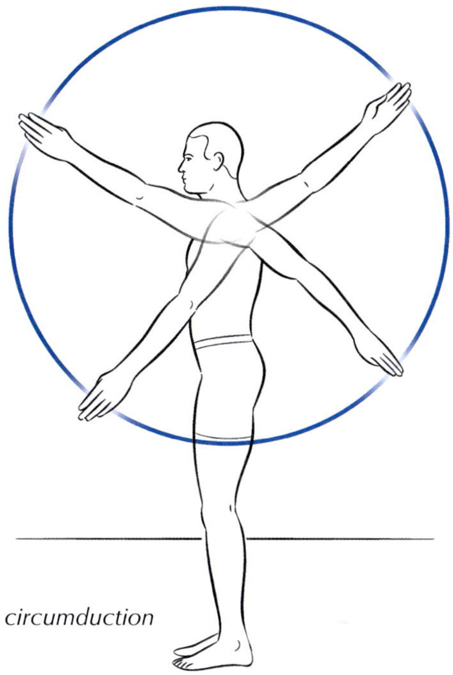

- *Shoulder circumduction*

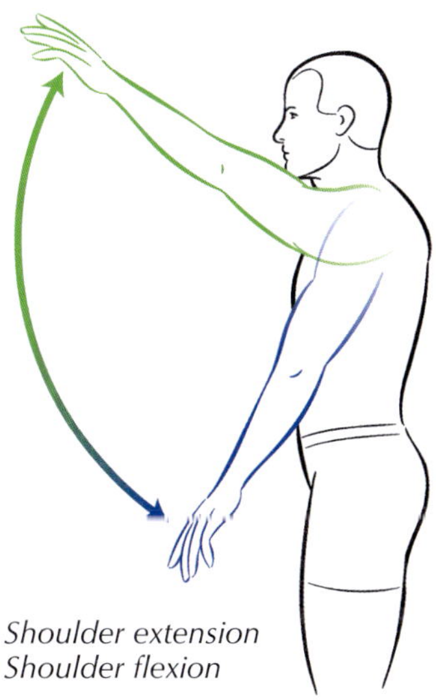

- *Shoulder extension*
- *Shoulder flexion*

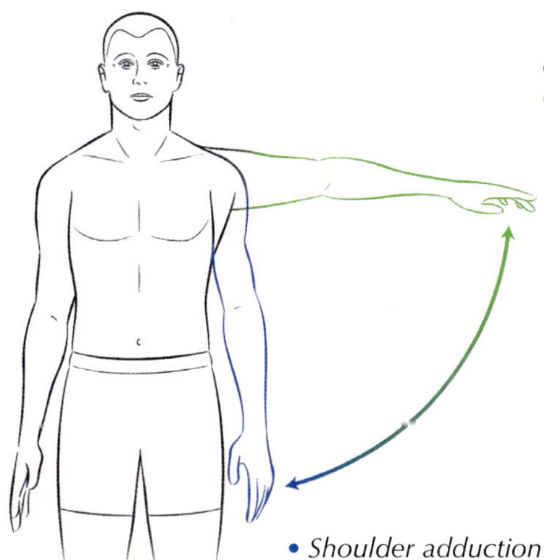

- *Shoulder adduction*
- *Shoulder abduction*

- *Elbow flexion*
- *Elbow extension*

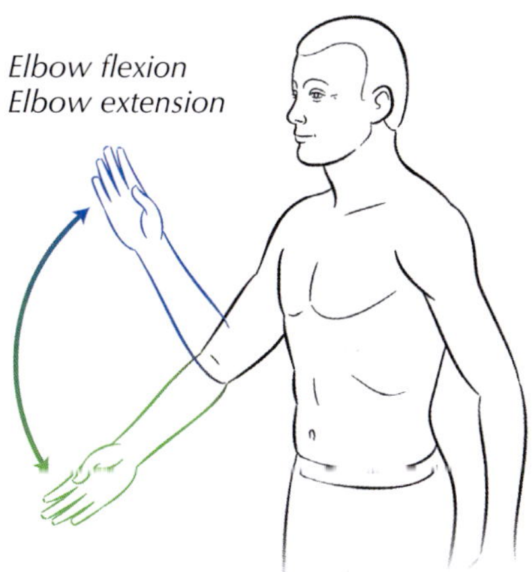

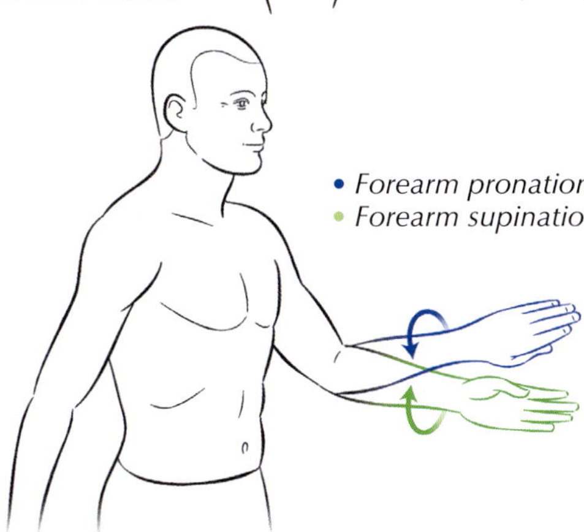

- *Forearm pronation*
- *Forearm supination*

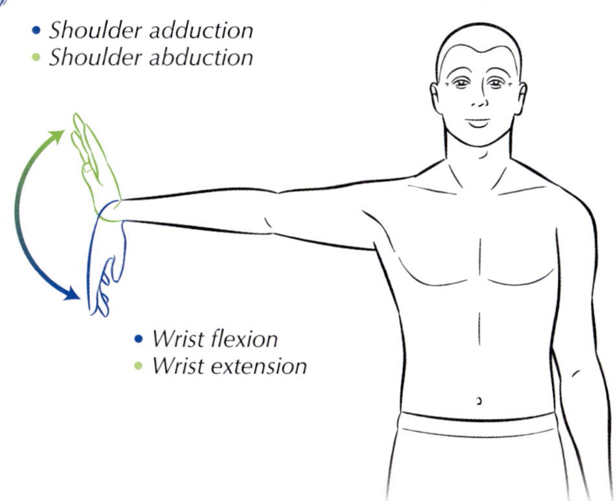

- *Wrist flexion*
- *Wrist extension*

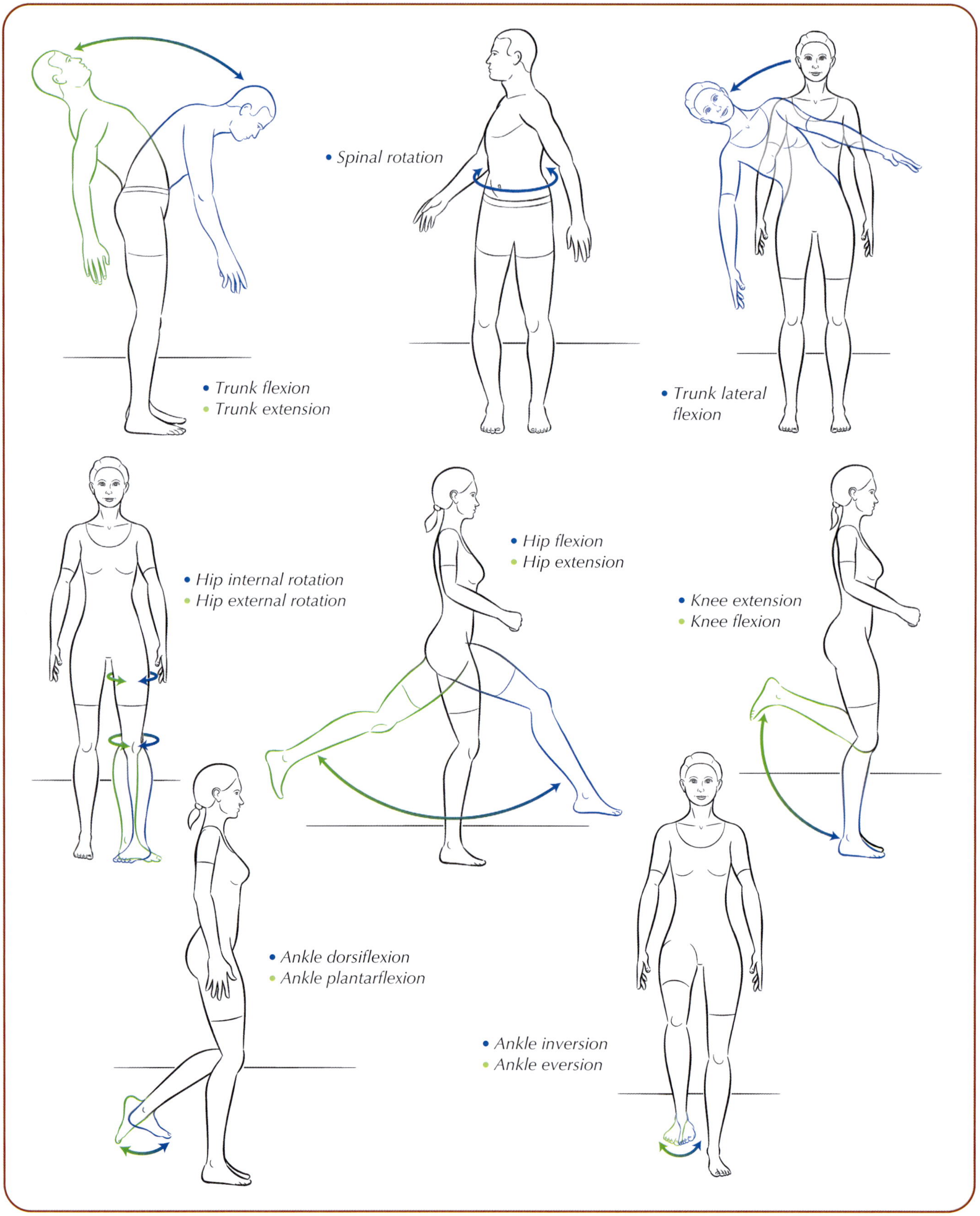

• Trunk flexion
• Trunk extension
• Spinal rotation
• Trunk lateral flexion
• Hip internal rotation
• Hip external rotation
• Hip flexion
• Hip extension
• Knee extension
• Knee flexion
• Ankle dorsiflexion
• Ankle plantarflexion
• Ankle inversion
• Ankle eversion

CLASSIFICATIONS OF INJURIES

Sprain

A sprain is a partial or complete tearing of a ligament. Sprains are caused when a joint goes through an excessive range of motion beyond its normal range. Severe sprains often occur with fractures and dislocations and when suspected should be referred for X-ray and medical attention. As ligaments are relatively avascular (having a poor blood supply), they take more time to heal than muscle tissue. The lack of blood supply makes it more difficult to get nutrients to the site to aid healing; it is also less capable of eliminating waste products. Swelling on a sprain is slower to emerge than for a strain. Swelling will take hours to develop on a sprain, whereas swelling on a strain would take minutes.

- **A first-degree sprain** is a minor tear of the ligament. Mild local pain and tenderness may be felt and minor swelling and muscle spasm may be seen. The function of the joint isn't too affected. With the correct treatment and care, recovery from a first-degree sprain can take about 2–3 weeks.
- **A second-degree sprain** is a severe partial tear of the ligament fibres. Pain may be experienced while at rest and is likely during weight-bearing and stress-testing. Considerable swelling and a loss of function are likely with this level of sprain. Recovery is likely to take about 3–6 weeks.
- **A third-degree sprain** is a total rupture of the ligament fibres. There will be severe pain, severe loss of joint function, loss of joint stability and muscular spasm. Rapid swelling is also likely around the joint. A possible pop can be heard if the incident is sudden or traumatic. Recovering from a third-degree sprain can take upwards of 3–4 months or more following surgery.

Strain

A strain is a tear in a muscle or tendon due to excessive tension through the tissue. Strains often occur at the musculotendinous junction. Muscle strains can often occur during heavy lifting or during explosive, fast movements, and at a time of muscular and neurological fatigue. Therefore, strains occur more often towards the end of sporting events. They can also be caused by an impact injury or compression. A poor warm-up by the athlete can increase the likelihood of a strain. As muscles and tendons have a better blood supply than ligaments and muscles have a greater blood supply than tendons, muscles tend to heal faster than tendons and tendons faster than ligaments.

- **A first-degree strain** is a minor partial tear. Some noticeable effect on function is likely to occur although is more likely during high intensity activity. Mild to moderate pain will be experienced during contraction and stretching. The strength of the muscle may be reduced with a possible tightening of the muscles, with potential swelling and tenderness with palpation. Recovery from a first-degree strain can occur very quickly.
- **A second-degree strain** is a severe partial tear. Function is impaired to a greater degree. Moderate to strong pain will be experienced during contraction, stretch and palpation. Muscle strength will be reduced and spasm of the affected and surrounding muscles is likely. Moderate to major swelling can occur and function will be greatly affected. Recovery from a second-degree strain may take 3–6 weeks with good treatment.
- **A third-degree strain** is a total rupture. This type of injury is due to a severe over-stretching or very forceful contraction. Athletes that may be at higher risk are Olympic weight-lifters, body builders and track-and-field sprinters. Signs and symptoms include severe pain (local and diffuse), loss of function, weakness, marked swelling, spasm in adjacent muscles and palpable bunching of the muscle fibres. This injury normally requires surgical intervention and can take 2–3 months or longer to recover.

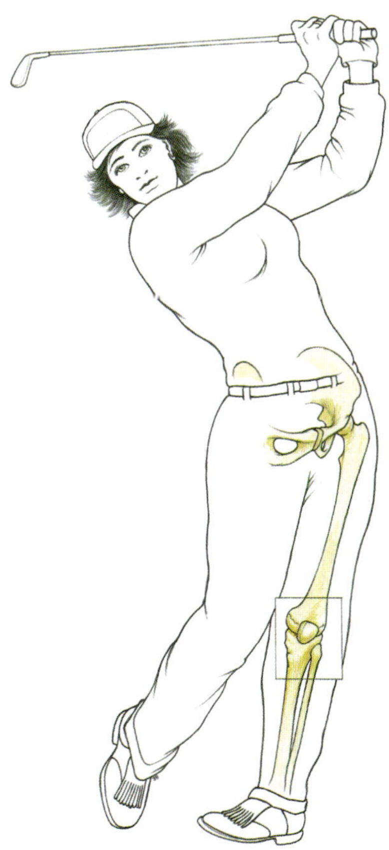

ACL sprain (see page 46).

Stress fractures

Stress fractures are hairline fractures of the bone, normally resulting as a consequence of repetitive physical stress. These fractures are most commonly suffered by long-distance runners, usually in the tibia or fourth or fifth metatarsal when the mileage is increased too quickly. Footballers, cricketers, throwers, ballet dancers and group exercise instructors are also vulnerable to this type of fracture.

The signs of a stress fracture are mild aching, local tenderness which is painful to press, swelling, pain decreasing with rest and increasing with activity, pain occurring earlier in workouts as the load is increased. These symptoms may not be too noticeable at first. They can then worsen with the aching becoming strong and distinct.

Stress fractures can be categorized either as *fatigue stress fractures* or *insufficiency stress fractures*. Fatigue stress fractures are the result of stress or overuse on normal bone. An insufficiency stress fracture is caused by normal stresses placed on abnormal bone.

Tendonitis

This painful condition is defined as an inflammation of a tendon. Tendonitis can occur with repeated stretching and overloading, causing the cross-linking structure of the collagen fibres to break apart, thus causing micro tears. These may be caused by tight muscles rubbing against a bone, ligament or retinaculum, external rubbing (for example, from a shoe), torsion and shear forces.

Due to the relative lack of blood supply to the tendons, they are slow to heal. Signs and symptoms of tendonitis include pain, tenderness and reduced strength. The symptoms often occur close to a joint, aggravated by activity as the lack of venous return can cause a long inflammatory period and build-up of nociceptive substances. Pain can often ease during activity and worsen after a period of rest.

Tenosynovitis, also known as tenovaginitis or paratendonitis, is the inflammation of the sheath that surrounds some tendons. Signs of tenosynovitis are crepitus (grating or crackling sounds) on movement, thickening of the tendon and fibrous adhesions inside the sheath. Common areas of tenosynovitis are the wrist and ankle.

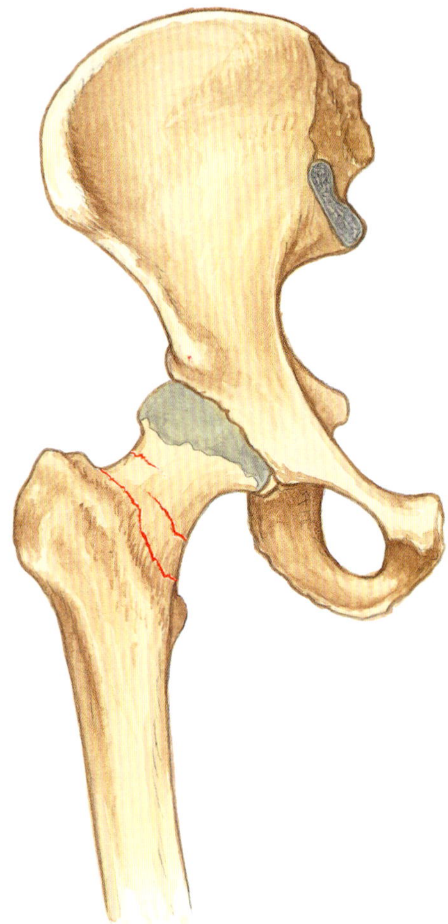

Stress fracture to neck of femur (see page 60 for more details).

Tissue healing times

Strain **First degree**-6 months	**Strain** **Second degree**	**Strain** **Third degree**
Days	3–6 weeks	2–3+ months
Sprain **First degree**	**Sprain** **Second degree**	**Sprain** **Third degree**
2–3 weeks	3–6 weeks	3–4+ months
Fractures	**Overuse Injuries**	
3–20 weeks	6 weeks	

INJURY PREVENTION
POSTURE AND MUSCLE BALANCE

Posture has become a quite a buzz-word in recent years. However, the understanding, importance and methods of correcting posture are often misunderstood. There are many definitions of posture including: 'The position from which the musculoskeletal system functions most efficiently' (Moshe Feldenkrais). In addition to the many definitions there are also two main categories of posture – static and dynamic.

Static posture

Static posture may be defined as 'the position of the body at rest, sitting, standing or lying' (P. Chek, *Golf Biomechanics Manual*). This means that if you have poor posture before you are moving, you are more likely to have poor posture while moving. Therefore, poor static posture will be expressed in your movements.

Dynamic posture

Dynamic posture may be defined as 'the ability to maintain an optimal instantaneous axis of rotation in any combination of movement planes at any time in space' (P. Chek, *Golf Biomechanics Certification Course Manual*).

As a simple analogy, you can think of your spine as an axis of rotation (like a crankshaft) and your arms as a means by which motion at the axis is expressed (like the connecting rod). If your spinal axis is faulty and expresses the exaggerated curvatures that go hand in hand with poor posture, your capacity to rotate efficiently will be significantly reduced. If your spinal axis is correctly aligned, you are far more efficient and are less likely to become injured.

Optimal posture is maintained when muscles surrounding a joint or joints are in balance. Good 'muscle balance' simply means that the muscles are at their optimal or normal length and tension. A muscle imbalance is when a muscle on one side of a joint is tight and its opposing muscle (antagonist) is long and potentially weak. This causes the joint to lose its optimal axis of rotation and can lead to excessive wear and tear on the joint and increase the likelihood for injury during physical activity.

It is beyond the scope of this book to instruct you on how to maintain optimal posture and muscle balance. Take advice from a qualified professional or read *Anatomy of Yoga for Posture and Health* by Brandon and Jenkins. It is always the goal of a rehabilitation programme to optimize posture and muscle balance.

Posture and alignment

The gravitational pull exerted on the body acts through the body in a straight line towards the centre of the earth.

In a standing position, neutral alignment occurs when body landmarks such as the ankles, knees, hips, shoulders and ears are in line with the pull of gravity. The body also requires balance from front to back and side to side, allowing it to maintain position against gravity with minimal effort. The more the body is out of alignment, the more energy it uses to resist the gravitational pull. For most athletes, poor posture will not only increase the likelihood of injury, it will also waste vital energy and could make the difference between winning and losing.

In neutral alignment, the pelvis is in a neutral position with the pubic ramus and the anterior superior iliac crest vertically aligned. In this position, if the pelvis was a bucket of water, no water would spill out. With an anterior pelvic tilt, the water would pour out the front and with a posterior pelvic tilt would cause the water to pour out the back.

As we exercise and move the body in different positions, for example when doing deadlifts or lunges, gravity continues to affect the body, the critical points of balance shift and we are required to work harder to maintain balance and alignment. Despite the fact that balance is shifting, when lifting heavy weights or jumping explosively, in some instances it is still important to maintain a neutral spine. 'Neutral spine' when performing deadlifts or jumping would require the maintenance of a straight line through the ear, shoulder, pelvis and hips, but not necessarily in a vertical line.

Poor postural control and alignment may affect your quality of movement and the safety and effectiveness of any exercise, as postural compensation is likely to occur. This means that the joints used, joint actions, range of movement and involvement of the various stabilizing and mobilizing muscles will change from the ideal, which will greatly increase the likelihood of injury.

EVENT PREPARATION

There is a big debate as to whether you should stretch before and/or after training and how you should warm up prior to workouts or competition.

There is evidence that suggests that stretching prior to exercise has no benefit and it can be detrimental to performance. There is some truth in these statements.

However, everything has to be carefully put into context with each individual situation. As noted on page 23, muscle balance and posture are crucial to optimizing performance and reducing the likelihood of injury. So here's my question. Do you want to train or compete with tight muscles and therefore poor muscular balance? Quite clearly, no!

So here's the deal. In rehabilitative, corrective or base conditioning phases of your training plan, corrective mobilizations and stretches are used to lengthen the short, tight and facilitated muscles in the body. These are normally the tonic muscles, but every individual is different. A simple way to check this is to perform stretches for each muscle group and if you feel tightness or discomfort in the targeted area, add it to your mobilizing and stretching programme. Ideally, you should seek a full assessment from a qualified professional, such as a CHEK practitioner, physiotherapist or strength and conditioning coach.

This pre-workout mobilization and stretching will allow the muscles to work through a wider range and for their antagonistic muscles to strengthen through a more optimal range without the risk of being inhibited.

As training becomes more intensive and moves into maximal strength, power or speed training, then this type of pre-stretching can be detrimental. If a muscle is stretched beyond its normal range or for too long, the nerve impulses that supply the muscles can be down-regulated. This means the muscles will produce less force.

Prior to maximal strength, rapid movements and competition, pre-event stretches and warm-ups should be performed. This is essential to prepare the bodily systems required prior to your workout or event in order to maximize your performance. By preparing the neuro-muscular system, cardiovascular system and respiratory system, you will be ready to perform at your best while minimizing the likelihood of injury. The possibility of injury is reduced because when muscles are warm, the tissues are less viscous and able to move through a wider range of motion and are therefore less likely to tear when moved quickly through a wide range at speed.

You should analyze the movement patterns of your sport or workout and use warm-up exercises that closely mimic those movements.

As you warm up, you should begin slowly and gradually increase the speed until you reach speeds close to that of your sport. By the end of your warm-up you should have a light sweat, but you should not over-do the warm-up and waste vital energy.

If you are in a phase of training using rapid movements, you should still perform corrective mobilizations and stretches. The only difference is when you perform them. You can perform them as part of your post event warm-down (cool-down) or prior to bedtime. This helps to remove metabolic waste from the muscles and anecdotal evidence suggests that stretching post-exercise helps to reduce muscle soreness.

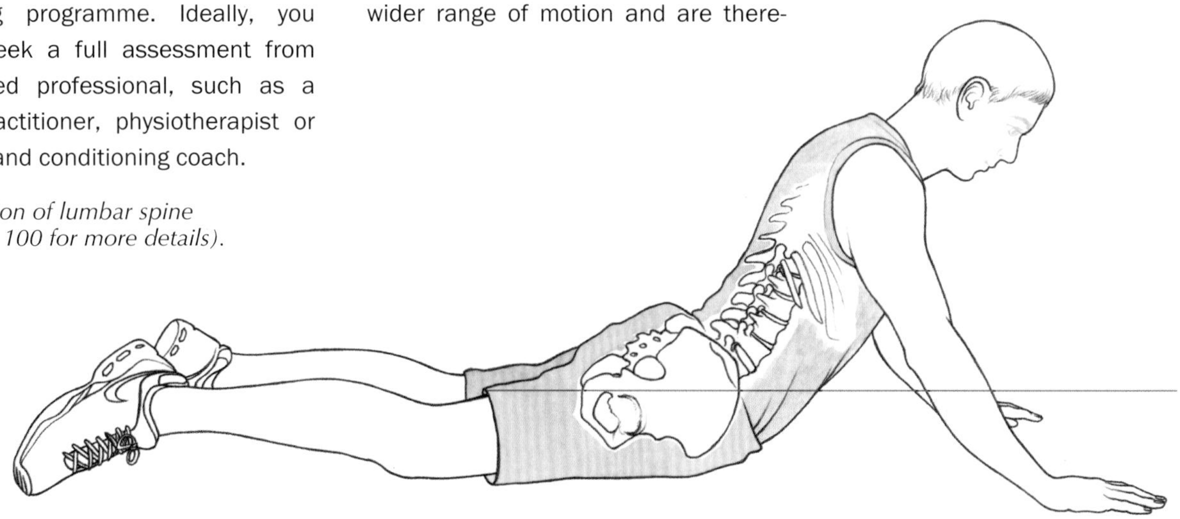

Mobilization of lumbar spine (see page 100 for more details).

RECOVERY

In order for performance to improve, you must train the body to go beyond its current capacity. In order to do so, the SAID principle needs to be understood. SAID stands for Specific Adaptation to Imposed Demands. What this means is that if you want to get stronger, you need to lift heavier loads than you currently can, or if you wish to increase endurance you need to run longer than you currently can at a given speed.

This is accomplished by training hard, beyond the level you have been training at and then allowing the body to adapt to the excess stress placed on it. So if you continually lift heavier weights the body will adapt to handle the stress under the right conditions. It will do this, for instance, by improving neural drive to the muscles, increasing muscle size etc. However, this will only occur if the body has adequate resources for the adaptations to occur. These resources include:

- Adequate rest and sleep
- Minimal stress (physical, mental and emotional)
- Adequate hormonal status
- Adequate nutritional status

With the correct conditions in place, training fatigue leads to an adaptation in the tissues and improved performance ability.

In order to ensure adequate recovery, a training and recovery diary should be kept which includes full details of the exercise programme, levels of muscle soreness, general energy/fatigue, ability to maintain technique and expected performance, body weight, appetite, resting heart rate, sleep patterns as well as levels of motivation, concentration and confidence. Signs of over-training include:

- Resting heart rate five beats per minute above or below normal (base)
- Unintentional or unexplained reduction in body weight of 3% or more
- Reduction in appetite
- Poor sleep quality for two days in a row or more
- Prolonged fatigue
- Muscle and bone soreness or joint ache
- Low motivation, attitude and confidence towards training.

So what can you do to optimize recovery?

- **Eat high-quality organic foods in accordance with your metabolic type®.**

Organic foods contain considerably more nutrients than non-organic foods and give your body the building blocks they need to recover. Eating right for your metabolic type® (see glossary page 141), allows for optimum function (including regeneration) of all cellular processes. Food provides the building blocks for your body's structures. If you eat a low-quality diet in the wrong proportions of macronutrients, you'll have weaker muscles, connective tissues and bones. You'll also have blood-sugar imbalances, causing a stress response in the body, which in turn leads to a reduction in growth hormone levels that are required for recovery and regeneration of tissues.

- **Remain fully hydrated.**

Most athletes will need a minimum of 0.03 litres (1.01 oz) of good-quality water per kilogram (2.2 lb) of body weight. For instance, a 50 kg (110 lb) woman would need a minimum of 1.5 litres (50 fl oz) per day. There are hundreds of thousands of biochemical reactions that take place in the human body every second and they all require adequate amounts of water.

- **Ensure adequate sleep.**

Adequate sleep means getting around 8–9 hours sleep per night and for elite athletes possibly 9–10 hours. Sleep times are crucial too – growth hormones in the body peak around 9.30 pm–10.30 pm and therefore it is essential that you are asleep by 10–10.30 pm each night to maximize your recovery. Our hormonal systems are tied into the movement of the sun (rise and fall) and going to bed late and getting up late will not compensate for missing the growth hormone window. Sleep in a totally dark room. Light hitting the skin has been shown to increase stress hormones, which are antagonistic to anabolic (growth) hormones.

- **Take passive and active rest days.**

Passive rest is when you take days off and do no physical activity whatsoever. These can be crucial when following very gruelling training mesocycles, preparing to peak or when the resting heart rate is five beats per minute above the base level.

Active rest is when you train, but at a lower intensity than normal or use a form of training that is different from your event or normal training routine. Active rest is often used post-event to aid the removal of metabolic waste from the muscles.

Rest days are crucial physiologically, psychologically and emotionally. An athlete should have at least one rest day per week.

Post-event or post-training recovery

Training and recovery diary

Name: Week commencing:

/ 10 / 10 / 10	Day 1	Day 2	Day 3	Day 4	Day 5	Day 6	Day 7
RHR (bmp)							
Time awoke							
Woke refreshed	Yes/No	Yes/No	Yes/No	Yes/No	Yes/No	Yes/No	Yes/No
Time asleep							
Breakfast							
Mid AM snack							
Lunch							
Mid PM snack							
Dinner							
Late snack							
Workout 1 **Intensity** **Volume**	H / M / L H/M/L	H / M / L H/M/L	H / M / L H/M/L	H / M / L H/M/L	H / M / L H/M/L	H / M / L H/M/L	H / M / L H/M/L
Workout 2 **Intensity** **Volume**	H / M / L H/M/L	H / M / L H/M/L	H / M / L H/M/L	H / M / L H/M/L	H / M / L H/M/L	H / M / L H/M/L	H / M / L H/M/L
Body weight	kg	kg	kg	kg	kg	kg	kg
Energy level	/ 10	/ 10	/ 10	/ 10	/ 10	/ 10	/ 10
Muscle soreness	/ 10	/ 10	/ 10	/ 10	/ 10	/ 10	/ 10
Joint aches	/ 10	/ 10	/ 10	/ 10	/ 10	/ 10	/ 10
Training attitude	/ 10	/ 10	/ 10	/ 10	/ 10	/ 10	/ 10
Training motivation	/ 10	/ 10	/ 10	/ 10	/ 10	/ 10	/ 10
Training confidence	/ 10	/ 10	/ 10	/ 10			

KEY:
RHR (Resting heart rate) to be taken in bed upon waking
Workouts: Record level of intensity as H = Hard, M = Medium, L = Light
Record level of volume as H = Hard, M = Medium, L = Light
Body weight to be taken first thing after using the toilet and before eating

should also include:

- A cool down, normally involving low-intensity exercise – light jogging, swimming or cycling – to aid the removal of metabolic waste from the tissues.
- Rehydration with good-quality mineral water to replace lost fluid.
- A meal or snack containing protein, fats and carbohydrates to replace lost nutrients. A meal or snack that is 10–15 percent higher in carbohydrates than normal will help to replenish muscle glycogen, as well as regeneration of muscle tissue.
- Ice bath or contrast shower to reduce inflammation of tissue damage and aid release of metabolic waste.
- Sports massage to help remove metabolic waste, relax the muscles, reduce muscular tone, release trigger points and improve digestive function. A massage is recommended at least once or twice per week.
- Meditation techniques can be very useful especially before bed. It helps stimulate growth hormones and aid repair and tissue regeneration.
- Stretching should be performed to prevent shortening of muscles and therefore avoiding sport-specific muscle imbalances. Stretching should be performed four hours after the event as metabolic waste continues to be released for up to four hours post exercise. Stretching should only be performed on tight or facilitated muscles, so a good understanding of your body's muscle balance is crucial.

Failure to recover adequately after exertion will greatly increase your likelihood of injury!

LONG-TERM REHABILITATION
TISSUE HEALING

There are three distinct stages in tissue healing: an acute inflammatory phase; a cellular proliferation phase; and a remodelling phase.

The acute inflammatory phase is the initial response to injury. In this phase you will find redness, swelling, heat, pain and impaired function. Swelling occurs due to bleeding from ruptured capillaries, vasodilation of the blood vessels in the local area, increased permeability of the vessels due to the release of histamine and other chemicals and flooding of fluid into the interstitial spaces around the injured area. The area is painful and tender due to an increase in tissue pressure and stimulation of pain receptors. Normal movement and function is inhibited due to the pain and swelling, which acts as a safety mechanism to avoid further injury. The main aim during this phase is to minimize inflammation. This phase lasts around three to five days.

The cellular proliferation phase is the early repair stage where the first series of structural repair begins. A new network of capillaries and lymphatics is developed which increases circulation and drainage. Then, specialized cells called fibroblasts are developed in the connective tissues. The fibroblasts produce the new ground substance of repair and the precursors of collagen, elastic and reticular fibres.

Collagen is the major component of bone, ligament, cartilage, tendon, skin, and scar tissue. Approximately five days after the injury, fibrous connective tissue is laid down, but it is still weak and vulnerable to re-injury. The strength of the tissues increases over the next three to four weeks as the capillary network decreases and the tissues strengthen with the formation of cross links in the collagen fibres.

Mobility exercises can begin during this phase within a pain-free range, but excessive stress on the tissues should be avoided. This phase lasts around two to five weeks.

The remodelling phase (also known as the maturation phase) is when the new tissue gains its strength through structural organization. With careful rehabilitation, the randomly arranged fibres become more organized and aligned along the lines of external stress placed on the tissues during normal activity and rehabilitation. During this phase, the rehabilitation becomes more aggressive with respect to mobilizations, stretching, proprioceptive work, strength and power, which prepare the tissues for the rigours of the sport. This phase usually lasts for several months.

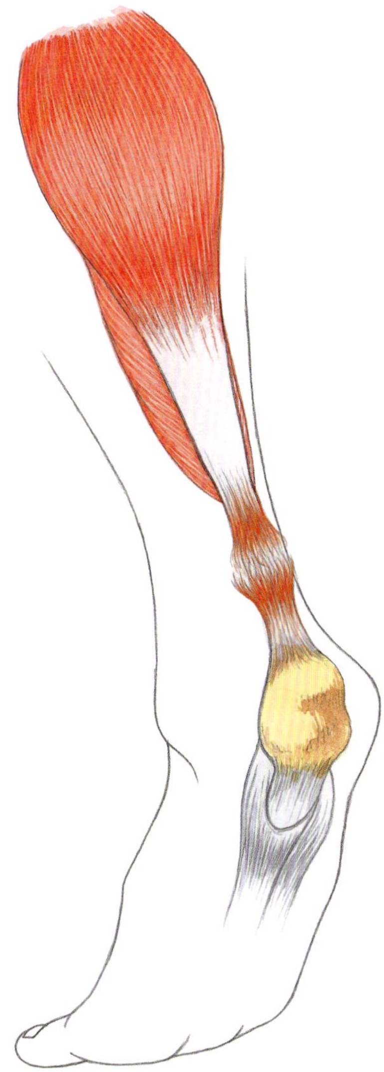

Acute inflammatory phase of Achilles tendonitis (see page 41 for more details).

LONG-TERM REHABILITATION
HEALING PHASES

Let's take a rehabilitation programme for a tennis player suffering an acute ankle sprain as an example:

Acute inflammatory phase

• RICE (Rest, Ice, Compression and Elevation, see page 29) of the ankle for the first 24–48 hours for 10–20 minutes every two hours; refer to a medical professional if a grade 3 sprain.

• Consume anti-inflammatory foods and supplements.

• A doctor may prescribe pain relief and anti-inflammatory medications or homeopathic anti-inflammatory ointments or injections such as Traumeel® can be used. Caution is urged since some anti-inflammatory medication can cause an inflammatory response in the gut and inhibit the abdominal musculature via viscero-somato reflex, making the lumbo-pelvic region more unstable and increasing the chance of future injury.

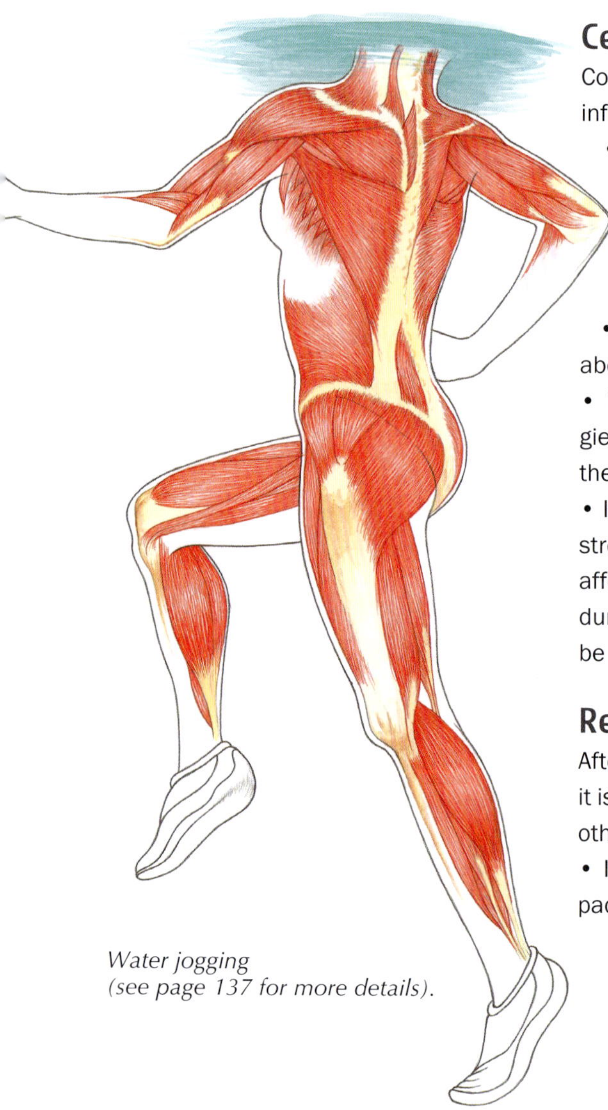

Water jogging (see page 137 for more details).

Cellular proliferation phase

Continue RICE as necessary. Once inflammation has subsided try:

• Passive movements of the ankle through a pain-free range of motion can be performed.

• Weight-bearing activities can begin if comfortable.

• Light sports massage (effleurage) above the ankle.

• Treatment of the potential aetiologies of the symptoms, e.g. muscles of the lumbo-pelvic region or lower limb.

• If the injury allows, begin upper-body strengthening, strengthening of the unaffected leg, general flexibility and endurance work. Strapping or taping may be useful during this stage.

Remodelling phase

After 3–5 weeks in the previous phase it is possible to move on to a number of other treatments and activities:

• Introduce heat such as saunas, hot packs, contrast baths and showers.

• Introduce deeper remedial massage techniques (petrissage, frictions, soft tissue release, positional release, neuromuscular therapy and muscle energy techniques) around the ankle.

• Hydrotherapy, such as walking and jogging in the pool can be introduced.

• Introduce stretching of the ankle.

• Proprioceptive and balance training can be introduced using wobble boards, stability discs and/or a BOSU®.

• Introduce strengthening exercises beginning with isometric contractions and progress to concentric and then eccentric contractions.

• Strapping or taping the ankle (in this particular case) may be useful during this stage.

Towards the end of the Remodelling phase, the athlete should progress through the continuum of flexibility, stability, strength and finally power before commencing competition. This will ensure end-stage rehabilitation and prevent a recurrence of the ankle injury or subsequent compensatory injury elsewhere in the body. This might include closed-chain exercises such as lunges, squats and deadlifts, standing cable pushes, pulls and rotations with increasing use of the legs to drive the movement.

A progression on to Olympic lifts, jump squats and jump lunges and dynamic medicine ball drills could be used to build power when enough strength has been built. A slow progression back into tennis could be introduced, increasing frequency, duration and intensity of sessions up to competitive levels.

ACUTE CARE – RICE

Acute injuries should be treated immediately with RICE (Rest, Ice, Compression and Elevation).

Rest should include stopping all activity to avoid further damage to tissues and to avoid further bleeding. Rest will also allow the re-alignment of damaged fibres to begin before any further damage is done. Rest includes no weight bearing, usually requires sitting or lying and no resisted movements for 48 hours to limit scar tissue.

Ice should be applied directly to the injured area through a wet cloth-like material (not directly onto the skin) to cool and reduce blood flow to the area and therefore reduce inflammation. Ice has also been shown to have an analgesic affect and can prevent associated muscle spasm and tension. The ice should be applied as soon as possible following the incident until the area just starts to go numb.

The affected area should be pale in colour when the ice is removed. If the area is red, it has been on too long. Icing an area for too long can reverse the process of preventing blood flow to the area and actually increase blood flow causing further inflammation. Areas such as the wrist may only require 5 minutes whereas an area such as the thigh may need as much as 20 minutes. It should then be removed until the area is back to normal temperature, by which time the ice can be re-applied. Ice can be applied as above for the first 7 days following the incident.

Compression should be applied to the injured area as soon as possible to minimize bleeding of the affected fibres as the compression of the blood vessels stops the bleeding. Compression should be performed with a firm pad held in place with strapping. Limbs should not be compressed all around to avoid restricting blood flow to the whole limb. Compression can be continued for a few days.

Elevation should be applied by keeping the affected area above the torso. This assists the flow of swelling away from the affected area. Any affected limb should be elevated and supported. Elevation should be applied as often as possible and used until all the swelling has gone.

FINDING THE CAUSE OF THE INJURY

When a part of the body is injured it is very easy to focus all the rehabilitative efforts on the site of the injury. While this may be crucial during the acute phase, it becomes less and less important and less effective as you move through the remodelling phase.

Think of it like this: you are rowing a boat and it springs a leak. Unless you do something quick, the boat will sink. Do you keep bailing out the water or do you plug the hole to stop the water coming in?

Plugging the hole gets to the cause of the problem whereas bailing out the water just deals with the effect of the leak. While we need to deal with the effect (the injury) at first, we need to understand the cause as well so that we can ensure the injury does not recur or cause a different injury in the future through a faulty recruitment pattern or compensatory pattern.

To ascertain the cause of injuries, for a number of years I have been using very successfully the Reflex Survival Totem Pole, something taught to me by Paul Chek, the founder of the CHEK Institute.

The Reflex Survival Totem Pole (right) highlights the systems of the body in a hierarchy dependent on each system's importance to human survival in the wild. Each system will be sacrificed to any higher system to ensure survival.

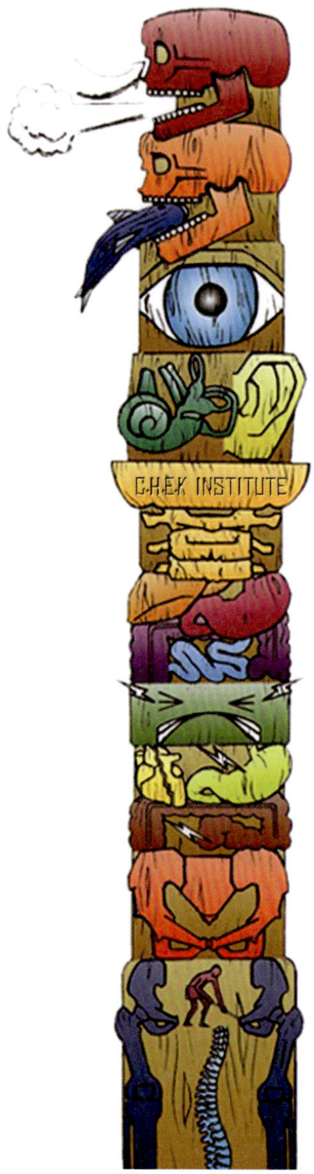

© CHEK institute, 2010

The systems in order are:

1 Breathing
2 Mastication
3 Vision
4 Vestibular (contributes to hearing, sense of balance and spatial awareness
5 Upper cervical spine
6 Viscera (internal organs)
7 Emotions and stress
8 Pelvic girdle
9 Slave joints

To give you a brief insight into the system, 'breathing' is at the top of the totem pole because it takes just three minutes without oxygen before brain cells begin to die. Therefore, the body will sacrifice everything else within the body to ensure respiration. Breathing can be affected by a restriction of air due to a blockage of the nasal passage for the following reasons:

- A short middle third (short nasal passage)
- Blocked nose (often caused by food sensitivities)
- Trauma to the face

To describe the Totem Pole in detail is beyond the scope of this book. However, I can state that I have tracked knee injuries to a malalignment of the upper cervical spine and ankle sprains to food sensitivities. The point is you have to understand that the human body is a system of interconnected systems and many times the connections are not always obvious. It is imperative that the cause or causes of any injury are found and remedied.

End-stage rehabilitation

The triangular diagram opposite illustrates how you need to periodize your whole rehabilitation programme from acute injury to end-stage rehab. Before you begin competition again, you must go through all the phases of training to optimize performance and prevent the recurrence of injury. Over the years, I have explained to my athletes and clients that to build a strong, stable, efficient body, you have to treat it like building a skyscraper.

Before you can construct any building, you need to provide solid foundations. This is also true for developing a body that is required to move quickly. Buildings need to be able to withstand earthquakes, extreme weather and other unforeseen stresses. Moving the human body at speed is similar to the stresses placed on a building during an earthquake. It has to handle a lot of stress without falling down.

With any construction, the stronger the foundations, the taller and stronger it can be. The same is true for the athlete. Therefore, we need to build strong foundations. A saying I find useful here is 'the wider the base, the taller the peak'. Therefore, it is important that a strong base of flexibility, stability and movement skill is achieved before moving to maximal strength, power and speed training.

Peak Performance Periodization

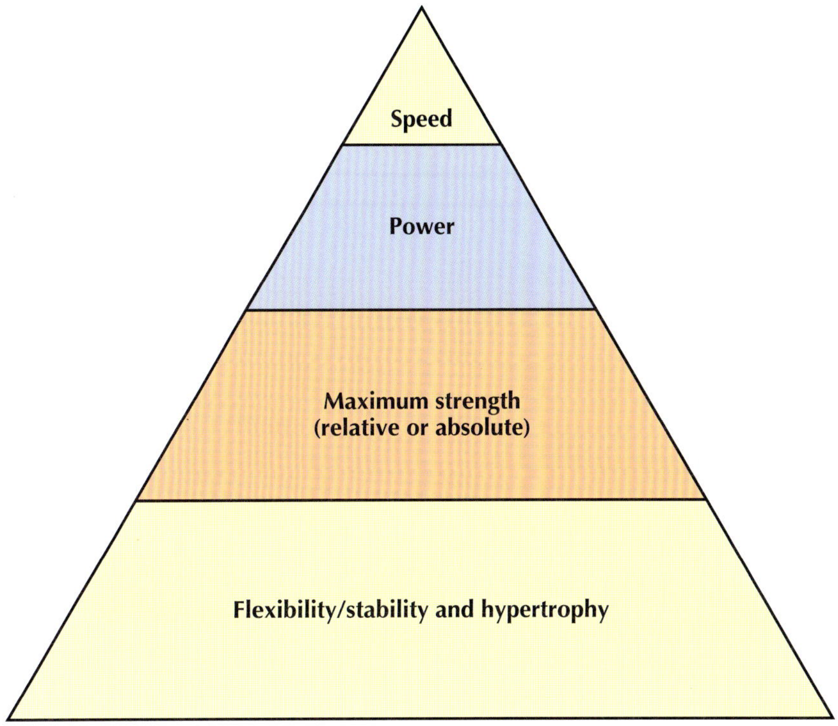

ANATOMY OF THE CORE

The 'core' is a real buzzword these days in the field of rehabilitation and performance. However, many talking about the core believe they are just referring to the abdominal musculature and perhaps the lower back. However, it's not that straightforward – the core is made up of 'inner' and 'outer' units.

Inner unit

The muscles of the inner unit of the core are the multifidus, pelvic floor, transversus abdominus and the diaphragm. These muscles create a 'cylinder-like' or 'corset-like' structure around the lumbar spine from the base of the ribs down to the pelvis, working together to stabilize the lumbar spine, the pelvis and the rib cage.

Stability of the spine, pelvis and rib cage are crucial to prevent injury and to provide a foundation for the limbs to create movement efficiently, powerfully and safely. The more stability created by the inner unit, the more power can be produced through the limbs and the likelihood of injury is reduced.

The inner unit muscles of the core should contract prior to the more superficial phasic muscles. Or to put it another way, the inner unit muscles contract to stabilize the lumbar spine, pelvis and rib cage prior to muscles of the outer unit. For instance, the transversus abdominus, pelvic floor and diaphragm have been shown to contract on average 30 milliseconds prior to an arm movement and 110 milli-seconds prior to a leg movement in all directions of limb movement. The outer unit muscles of the trunk contract later than the inner unit muscles. The timing of contraction of outer unit trunk muscles is dependent on the direction of movement of the limb. The difference between the inner unit muscles of the core is that they are controlled by the central nervous system independently of the outer unit trunk muscles. It has also been shown that when one muscle of the inner unit contracts, the other muscles of the inner unit also contract. This suggests that these muscles are on the same neurological reflexive loop.

The muscles of the inner unit of the core have shown that they can be inhibited due to pain or reflex inhibition, sensory-motor amnesia and viscero-somato reflex. In simple terms, pain in the abdominal region or lumbar spine, a lack of physical activity or inflammation of an internal organ can cause these inner-unit muscles to be inhibited and unable to contract normally. This leaves the spine exposed, increases the likelihood of injury and reduces the amount of power available.

There are many different views amongst experts with regards to training the inner unit. Some suggest not consciously focussing on it at all and suggest just stiffening all the abdominal muscles, known as 'bracing', to stabilize the spine. This technique does have its place and does help to increase stability in healthy individuals. However, in instances where the inner-unit muscles may be inhibited, bracing may not be effective because it is the inner-unit muscles that provide segmental stability of the spine. An inability to stabilize an individual spinal segment of the spine during a heavy lift could expose the spine to uncontrolled shear or torsion (see glossary page 141) and result in serious injury. Also, the bracing technique can also limit rotation of the torso. Rotation of the torso is used in most movements in sport. Bracing while rotating the torso is like driving your car with the hand-brake on! You waste energy and limit the amount of rotation.

In my clinical practice I have found a technique that works, taught to me by Paul Chek, the founder of the CHEK Institute. It involves using a conscious focus on inner unit contraction in an isolated environment (Four-point Tummy Vacuum page 115) when someone has a dysfunctional inner unit. This exercise allows the athlete to contract the muscles consciously without having to think about other muscle movements. As the athlete becomes confident with the muscular contraction, the exercises can be progressed to include coordination with outer unit muscles. The horse stance position (page 122) is particularly effective as the viscera create a stretch and excite the muscles spindles (see glossary page 141) of the transversus abdominus muscle, which increases its ability to contract. Also, the horse stance position, when performed correctly, creates a neutral spine position, from which more muscle fibres of the transversus abdominus are able to contract.

Ultimately, you will be required to integrate contraction of the inner unit muscles with your outer unit muscles subconsciously from a standing position (if your sport is performed standing up). It is advised that you complete inner unit exercises at the end of gym workouts to ensure you do not fatigue the stabilizer muscles prior to completing large compound movements (see glossary page 141).

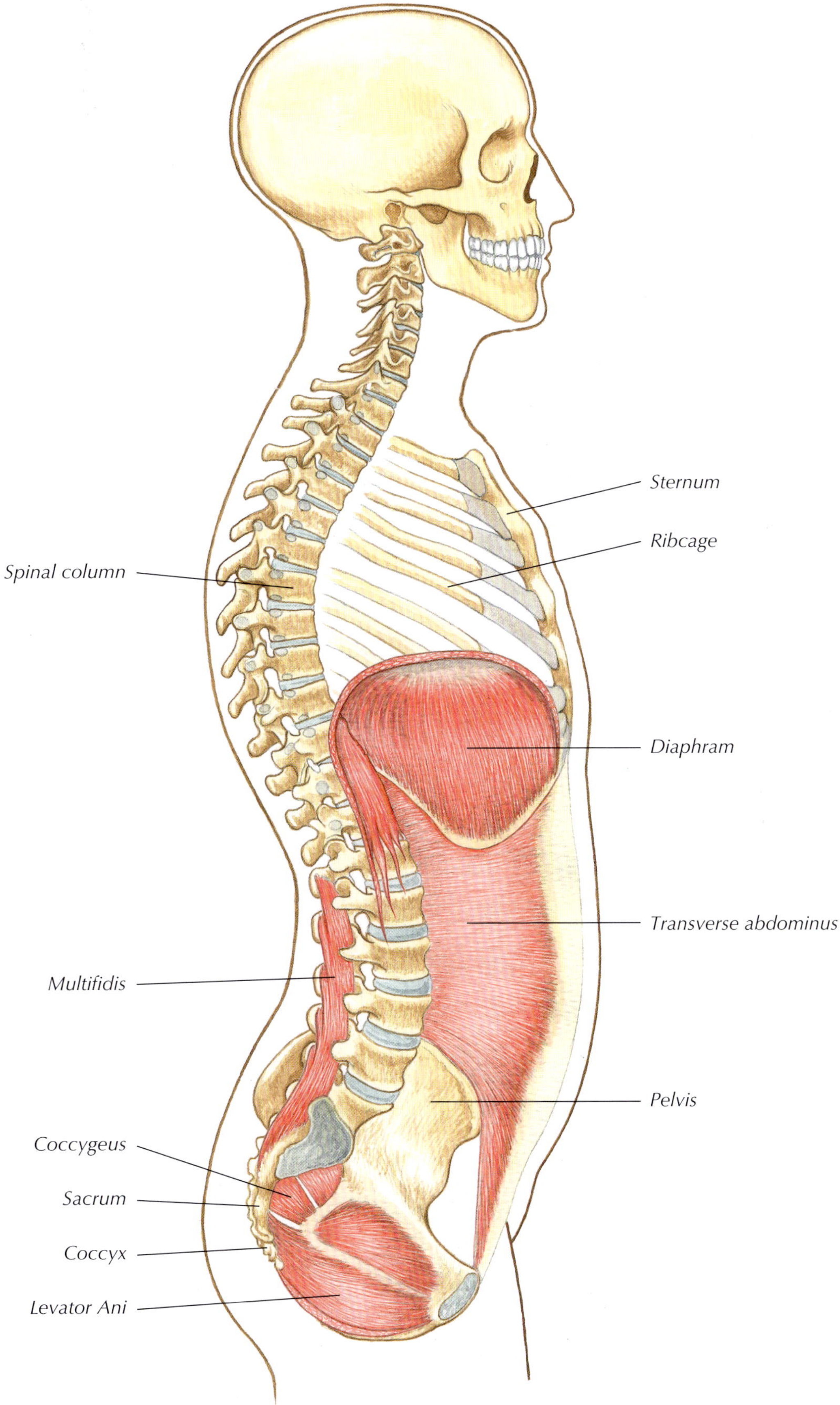
Sternum
Ribcage
Spinal column
Diaphram
Transverse abdominus
Multifidis
Pelvis
Coccygeus
Sacrum
Coccyx
Levator Ani

Outer unit

The 'outer unit' of the core is made up of four distinct systems: the anterior oblique, posterior oblique, lateral and deep longitudinal systems. The outer unit has a dual role in that it helps the inner unit to stabilize and it is also required to generate movement. Whereas the inner-unit muscles are tonic in nature (stabilizers), the outer unit muscles are generally phasic (mobilizers).

Anterior oblique system

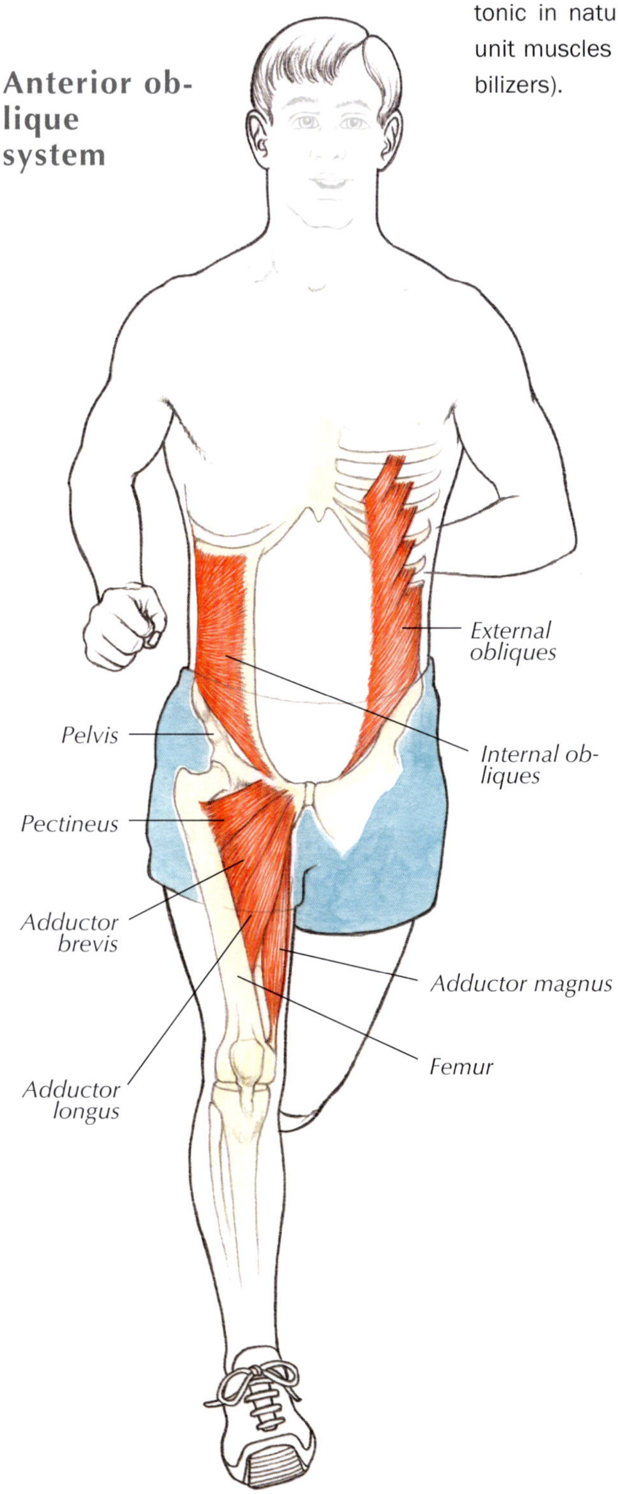

Posterior oblique system

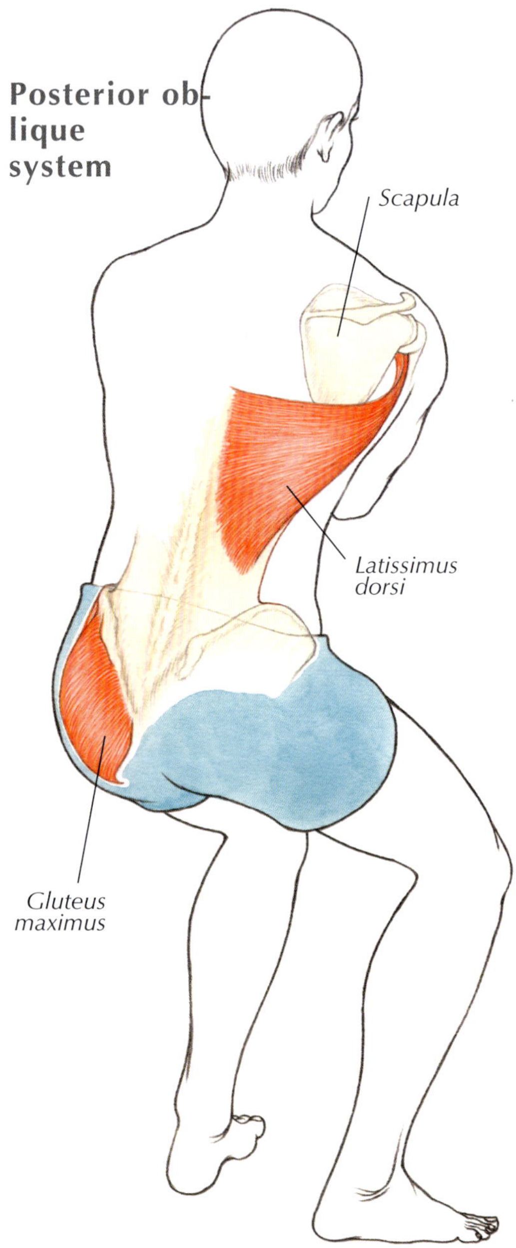

The outer unit systems work in conjunction with each other to:

- Create rotation in the torso and pelvis during gait.
- Help to stabilize the torso above the stance leg in gait and allow for optimal positioning of the heel for heel strike.
- Play a significant role in many sporting movements.
- Propel the body forwards during the propulsive phase of gait.
- Stabilize the sacroiliac joint of the stance leg during gait.
- Reduce the energy requirement for gait, therefore improving efficiency.
- Stabilize the torso above the stance leg during gait.
- Create stability through the sacro-iliac joint prior to heel strike through form and force closure.
- Slow down hip flexion and knee extension during the late swing phase gait.
- Stabilize the foot and ankle at heel strike.
- Aid rotation of the spine and reduce the energy cost of gait.

To summarize, effective inner and outer units of the core are required to minimize injury and optimize movement and performance. It is beyond the scope of this book to describe how to do outer-unit exercises, but they can be found by reading *Anatomy of Strength and Fitness Training for Speed and Sport* by Brandon.

Deep longitudinal system

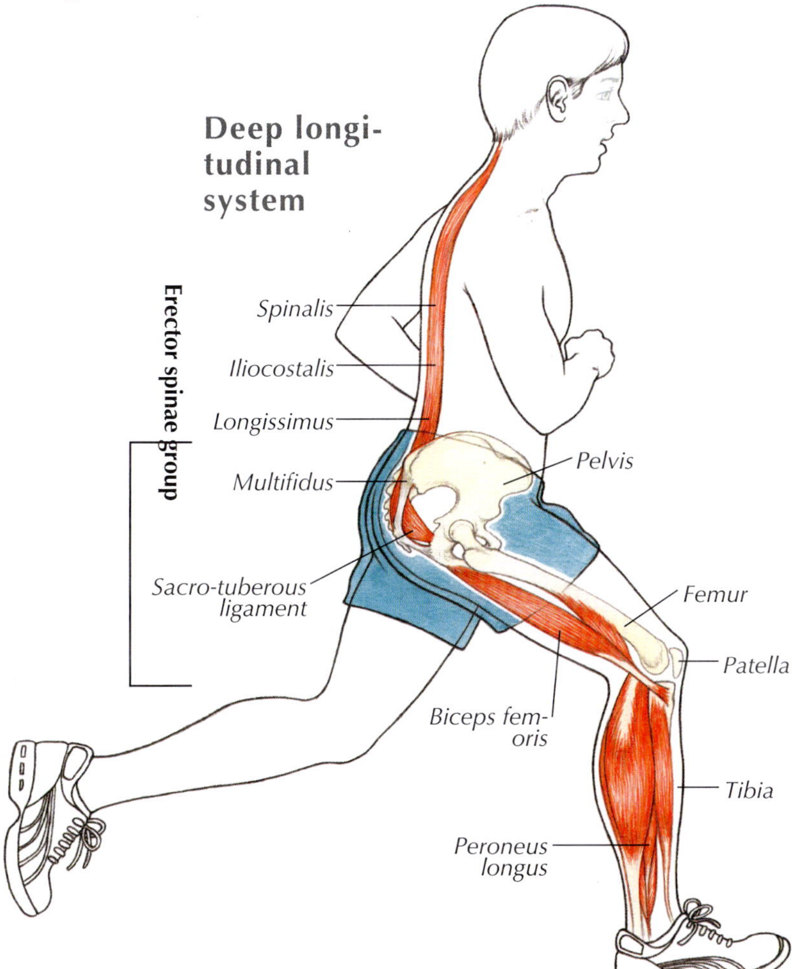

Lateral system

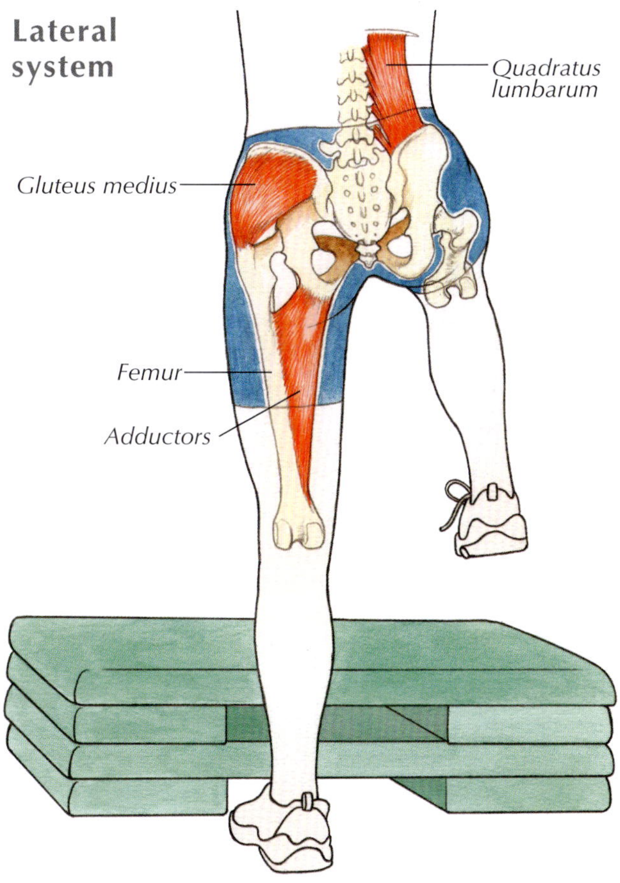

DESIGNING YOUR PROGRAMME

Before designing your rehabilitation programme, there are a number of factors that you need to take into consideration.

Exercise variables

Exercise variables are the loading parameters used during each lift or exercise in a training session. Exercise variables include the speed of movement (tempo), repetitions completed, rest period between sets and the intensity, which is often measured in terms of percentage of a one repetition maximum (1 RM)).

Initially, strength training should start at very low intensities, slow tempos and short rest periods. Isometric strength should be developed first, then concentric and finally eccentric strength.

As the tissues strengthen, intensity can be increased, tempo of movement can be increased and rest periods will need to be longer. For more details on exercise variables see *Anatomy of Strength and Fitness Training for Speed and Sport* by Brandon.

Open- versus closed-chain exercises

In human movement and therefore in sport, movements can be classified as open-chain or closed-chain.

Open-chain movements occur when the part of your body overcomes a load, be it gravity, a bat, a ball, an opponent, a weight etc. For example, if your sport involves throwing a ball or a punch, your body and arm are able to overcome the load of the ball, gravity and air resistance to launch through the air. If your sport requires you to kick a ball or an opponent, the same philosophy applies for the kicking leg.

Closed-chain movement occurs when you are unable to overcome a load and you pull or push yourself across the object. For instance, a rock climber will push with the legs and pull with the arms to climb up a rock face. The rock climber cannot overcome the rock face, but can move across it. Closed-chain movements also occur when you are walking and running. When running your propulsive leg drives into the ground and propels you forwards. You aren't able to make the ground move, but you do move across the ground.

For your sport you need assess whether you use open- and/or closed-chain movements and in what proportions. You can then choose the correct exercises to condition your body effectively for your sport. For most sports, the upper body requires a predominance of open-chain exercises and the lower body requires closed-chain exercises.

For many injuries, especially lower limb and shoulder injuries, it is often safer and more effective to begin strength training exclusively in a closed-chain environment.

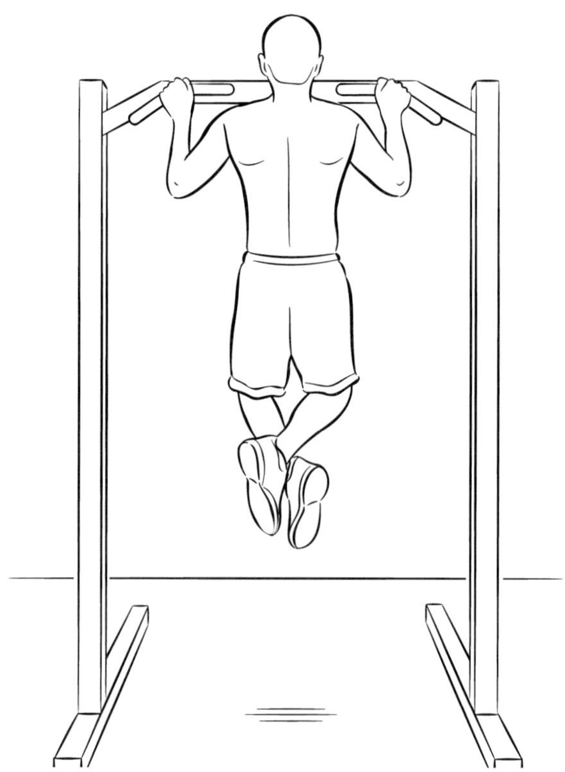

Upper body closed-chain exercise

Planes of motion

It is also crucial that tissues are strengthened in all planes of motion. Most injuries occur in the transverse and frontal planes. This is possibly due to a dominance of sagittal plane strengthening and therefore a lack of transverse and frontal plane conditioning. Therefore, you should analyze your sport and determine what proportion of each plane of motion is required for your sport.

For instance, rowers have a predominance of sagittal plane, with a tiny amount of transverse plane, whereas a golfer has a predominance of transverse plane movement and frontal and sagittal plane stability. Failure to condition tissues in all three planes is likely to lead to a return to the treatment table.

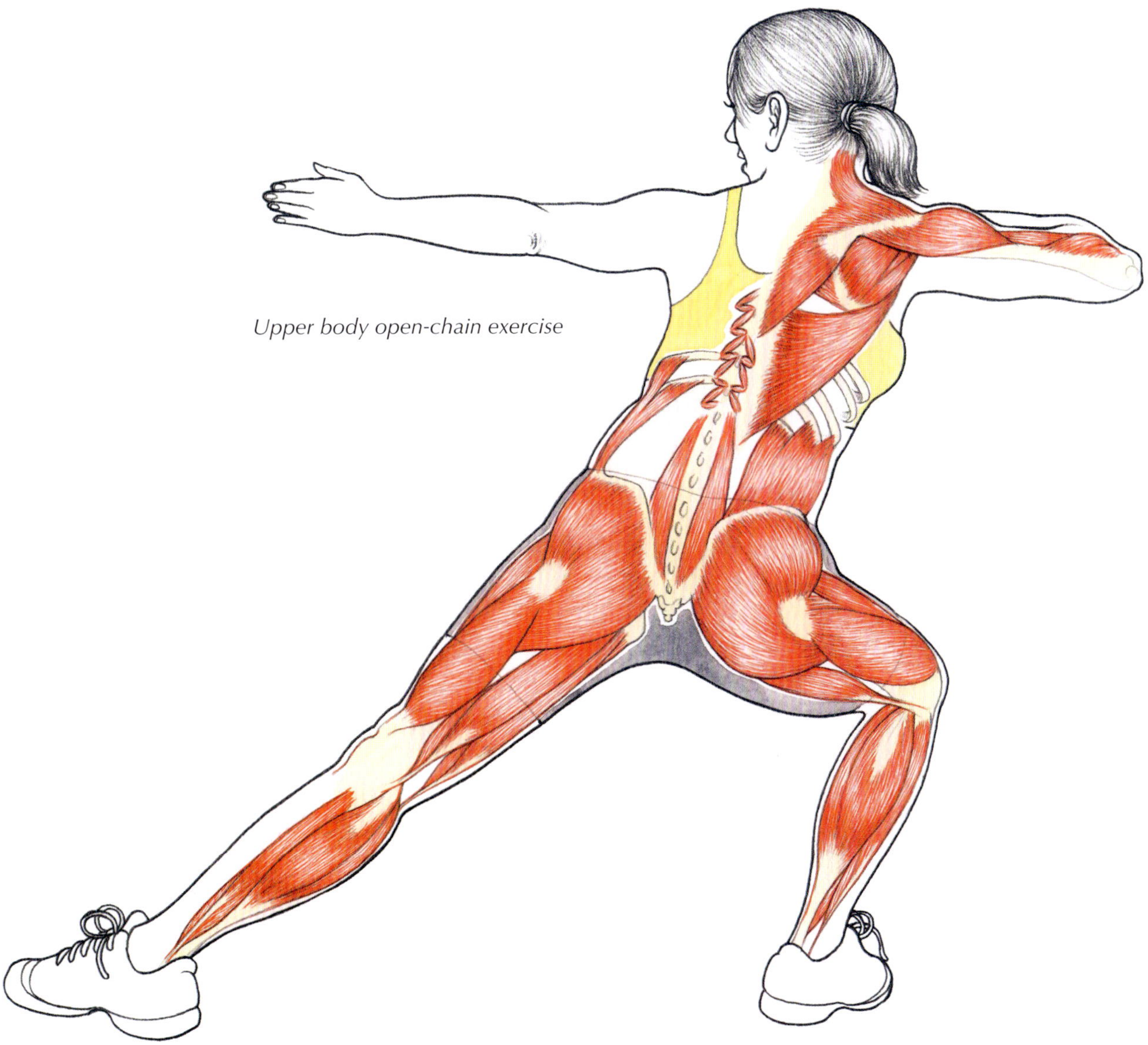

Upper body open-chain exercise

PART 2 COMMON SPORTS INJURIES

FOOT INJURIES

HALLUX VALGUS

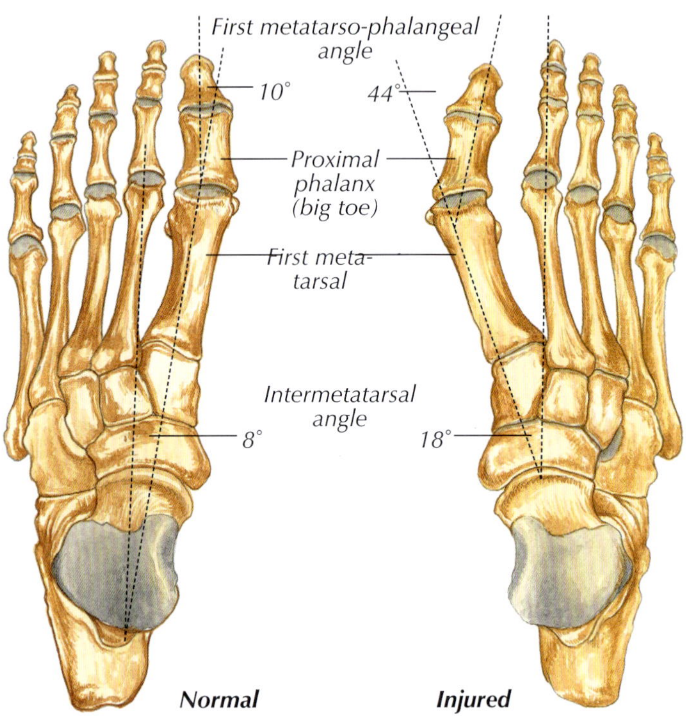

Description

This particular injury is in fact a structural anomaly where the first metatarsophalangeal joint moves inward towards the second toe. A hallux valgus often leads to a bunion, a bony lump on the side of the foot. Bunions are more prevalent in women than men, and some 2 million people were reported as having bunions in the USA in 2003, approximately 1 in 51 people.

Symptoms

- A bunion can eventually cause discomfort and pain.
- The skin over the lump can become red, blistered or infected.
- A fluid-filled space called a bursa may also develop under the skin in this area and this can cause pain if it becomes inflamed.

Causes

- High-heeled or pointed shoes.
- Over-pronation in the affected limb.
- Core instability (possible visceral inflammation).
- A lower cross syndrome.

Treatment

- Correct footwear. Wear well-fitting shoes with enough room to wiggle your toes, preferably shoes without a high heel.
- Corrective exercise to prevent a gravity pattern
- Strength training normally begins with isometric, then concentric and finally eccentric work is added.
- May require surgery in severe cases.

Exercises

Stretching

- Any tight muscles around the hip, knee or ankle joints should be stretched within pain-free ranges. These will differ from person to person.

Strengthening

- Strengthen the following muscles: gluteus maximus, gluteus medius and minimus, transversus abdominus and external obliques.

See exercises
- *Four-point tummy vacuum (page 115)*
- *Adductors (page 105)*
- *Lunge (page 128)*

RECOVERY TIME WITH APPROPRIATE RECOVERY MANAGEMENT
Between 3 and 6 months
after surgery

METATARSAL FRACTURE

Description

The five metatarsal bones are located between the tarsal bones of the hind-foot and the proximal phalanges. The metatarsals play a major role in support and propulsion. Fractures normally occur due to trauma, excessive rotational forces or over-use. The injury can result from participation in most sports.

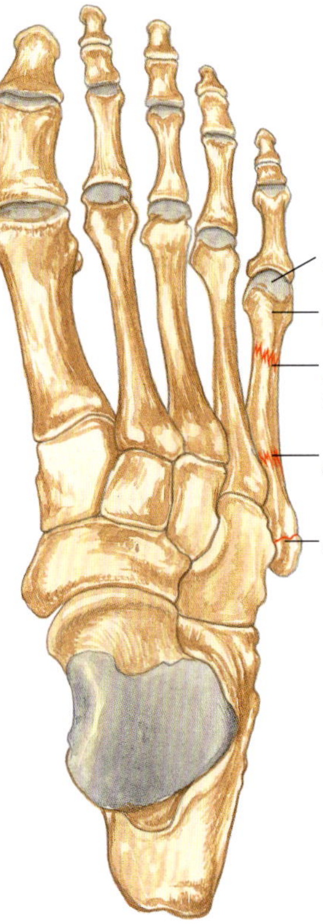

Symptoms

- Severe pain in the mid-front foot comes on gradually.
- Inability to bear weight due to pain.
- Painful to touch the region of the fracture.
- Swelling and bruising after a day or two.

Causes

- Impact injuries, such as kicking the underside of a football (soccer) boot.
- Poor landing with a twisting of the ankle.
- Over-use, such as an overly aggressive increase in mileage of a distance runner, commonly affecting the second, third or fourth metatarsals and is commonly seen in runners and gymnasts.
- Stress injuries may be caused by a gravity pattern.

Treatment

Acute

- If a fracture is suspected, a visit to the accident and emergency unit should be sought to receive an X-ray.
- In the first 24 to 48 hours, use RICE (see page 29) to prevent further damage and optimize healing time.
- An ankle cast is normally given to immobilize the area, plus the intermittent use of ice.
- Surgery is sometimes used to improve healing times to fractures of the base of the fifth metatarsal.

Post-acute

- Slow and gradual increase in activity and training. Stress fractures may require strengthening of the muscles that control lower limb pronation.

RECOVERY TIME WITH APPROPRIATE RECOVERY MANAGEMENT
May take 6 to 12 weeks

Exercises

Stretching

- Mobilization of the ankle joint in pain-free ranges should be used as early as possible to regain range of motion of the ankle joint.

Strengthening

- Once weight-bearing is possible and inflammation has ceased, strengthen the following muscles to prevent recurrence of stress fracture: gluteus maximus, gluteus medius and minimus, transversus abdominus and external obliques.

See exercises
- *Stand/squat on balance board (page 124)*
- *Four-point tummy vacuum (page 115)*
- *Lunge (page 128)*

PLANTAR FASCIITIS

Description

The plantar fascia originates from the tuberosity of the calcaneous and attaches to the metatarsal heads and the base of the five proximal phalanges of the foot. It is a thick fibrous band of connective tissue that supports the longitudinal arch of the foot. Plantar fasciitis is an inflammatory condition, but often presents with degenerative changes and therefore could be called plantar fasciosis. This injury accounts for between 5 and 14% of all running injuries in the USA. It is not gender-specific and occurs in athletes and non-athletes alike.

Symptoms

- Pain is often felt at its origin on the medial tubercle on the calcaneous, which can also radiate along the plantar fascia.
- Pain is most notable in the morning, symptoms often ease, but then increase throughout the day and with increased or prolonged activity.

Causes

- Lack of ankle dorsi-flexion secondary to tight gastrocnemius and/or soleus.
- Hallux limitus, which is a lack of extension of the big toe.
- Over-pronation (known as a gravity pattern) in the affected limb. This can be caused by weak gluteus maximus, gluteus medius and abdominal musculature and/or a lower-cross syndrome.

Treatment

Acute

- RICE (see page 29).
- Night splints and/or taping.

Post-acute

- Massage or self massage (self myofascial release).
- Corrective exercise.
- Strength training normally begins with isometric, then concentric and finally eccentric work is added.
- Anti-inflammatory protocols.

Exercises

Stretching

- The gastrocnemius and soleus muscles should be stretched gradually to improve ankle dorsiflexion.

Strengthening

- Strengthen the following muscles: gluteus maximus, gluteus medius and minimus, transversus abdominus and external obliques.

RECOVERY TIME WITH APPROPRIATE RECOVERY MANAGEMENT
1 week to several months

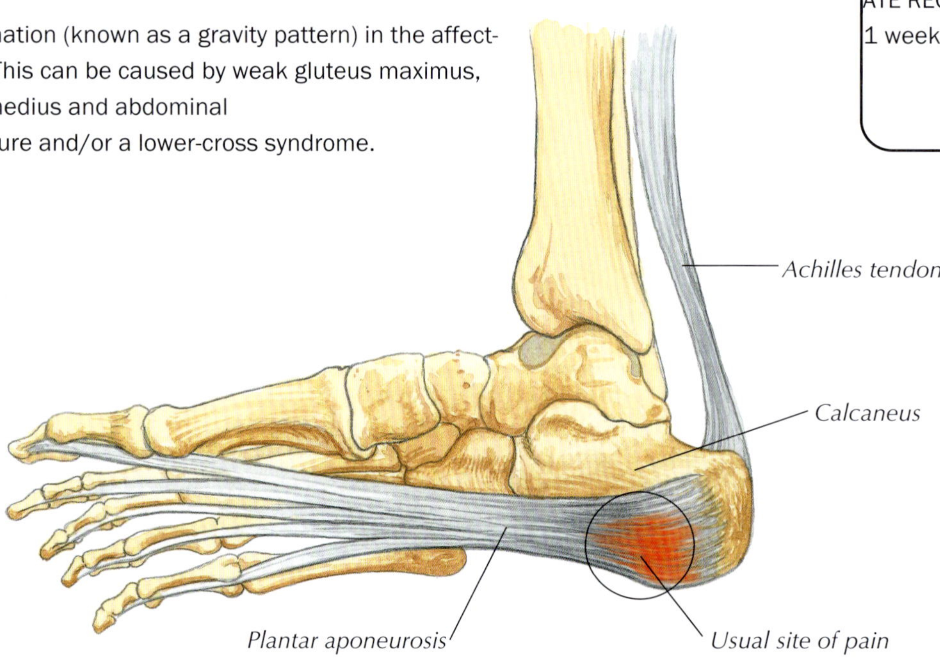

See exercises
- Calf stretch (page 107)
- Four-point tummy vacuum (page 115)
- Lunge (page 128)

ANKLE AND SHIN INJURIES

ACHILLES TENDONITIS

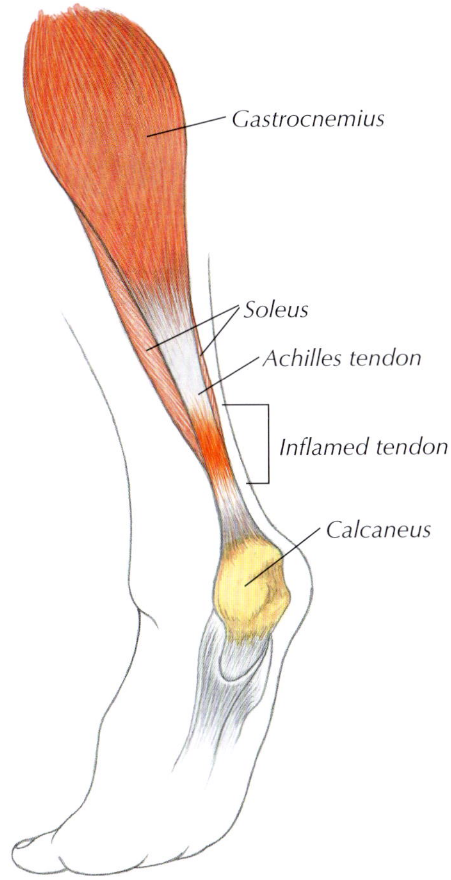

Description

Achilles tendonitis is an inflammation of the achilles tendon. The Achilles tendon is also known as the calcaneal tendon. It joins the gastrocnemius and soleus muscles to the calcaneous. Achilles tendonitis is more often referred to as Achilles tendinopathy since degeneration normally exists. It accounts for 11% of all running injuries and is more likely in athletes who spend a lot of time jumping, such as in basketball and volleyball.

Symptoms

Acute tendonitis

- Gradual onset of pain over a 2 to 3 day period.
- Pain at the onset of exercise which then fades during exercise.
- Pain eases with rest.
- Tender to touch.

Chronic tendonitis

- Gradual onset of pain over several weeks or months.
- Constant pain with exercise, especially going uphill.
- Pain and stiffness in the Achilles tendon especially in the morning or after rest.
- Nodules may be found in the tendon, approximately 2–4 cm (1-2 inches) above the heel.
- Tender to touch.
- Swelling or thickening over the Achilles tendon
- Possible redness over the skin.

Causes

- Over-pronation in the affected limb.
- Core instability (possible visceral inflammation).
- A lower cross syndrome.
- Tight calf muscles.
- Excessive heel cushioning (increasing the stretch on the tendon during running).
- Over-training.
- Excessive increase in training, especially uphill running.

Treatment

Acute

- In the first 24 to 48 hours, use RICE to prevent further damage and optimize healing time.

Post-acute

- Taping.
- Sports massage.
- Corrective exercise, leading to gradual return to training and competition.
- Correct footwear.
- Strength training normally begins with isometric, concentric and finally eccentric work is added.
- Total rupture requires surgery.

RECOVERY TIME WITH APPROPRIATE RECOVERY MANAGEMENT
3 weeks to 3 months

See exercises
- *Calf stretch (page 107)*
- *Squat on balance board (page 124)*
- *Lunge (page 128)*

Exercises

Stretching

- Gradual stretching of the gastrocnemius and soleus muscles
- Any tight muscles around the hip, knee or ankle joints should be stretched within pain-free ranges. These will differ from person to person.

Strengthening

- Once weight-bearing is possible and inflammation has ceased, strengthen the following muscles: gastrocnemius, soleus, gluteus maximus, gluteus medius and minimus, transversus abdominus and external obliques.

ACHILLES TENDON RUPTURE

Description

Achilles tendon rupture is a total rupture of the Achilles tendon. The Achilles tendon is also known as the calcaneal tendon. It joins the gastrocnemius and soleus muscles to the calcaneous. This injury most commonly occurs in older male recreational athletes.

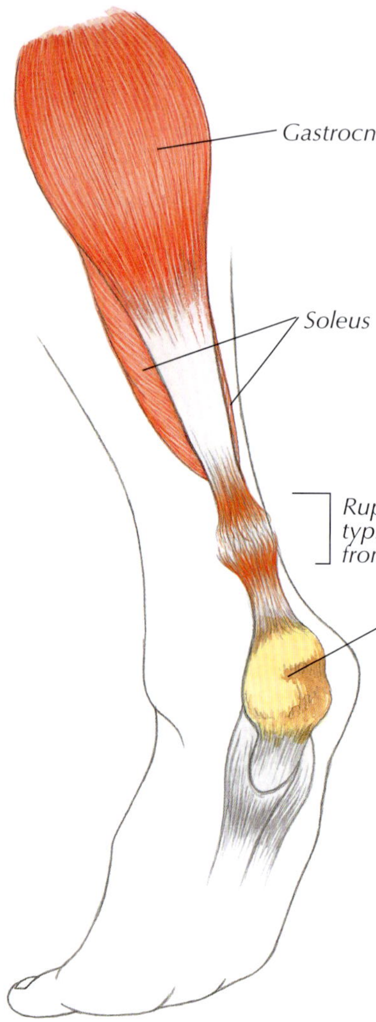

RECOVERY TIME WITH APPROPRIATE RECOVERY MANAGEMENT
6 weeks to 12 months

Symptoms

- Extreme sudden pain.
- Often a loud ‘pop’ or ‘crack’ is heard.
- Inability to weight bear or walk.
- Swelling.
- Bunching of the calf muscles towards the knee.

Causes

- A rapid change in contraction of the calf muscles from eccentric to concentric.
- Over-pronation in the affected limb.
- Core instability (possible visceral inflammation).
- A lower cross syndrome.
- Occurs often in sprinting-type movements, especially in untrained individuals.

Treatment

Acute

- A total rupture usually requires surgery
- In the first 24 to 48 hours, use RICE to prevent further damage and optimize healing time.

Post-acute

- Taping.
- Sports massage.
- Corrective exercise, leading to gradual return to training and competition.
- Strength training normally begins with isometric, then concentric and finally eccentric work is added.
- Correct footwear.

Exercises

Stretching

- Gradual stretching of the gastrocnemius and soleus muscles.
- Any tight muscles around the hip, knee or ankle joints should be stretched within pain-free ranges. These will differ from person to person.

Strengthening

- Once weight bearing is possible and inflammation has ceased, strengthen the following muscles: gastrocnemius, soleus, gluteus maximus, gluteus medius and minimus, transversus abdominus and external obliques.

See exercises
- *Calf stretch (page 107)*
- *Squat on balance board (page 124)*
- *Lunge (page 128)*

ANKLE SPRAIN

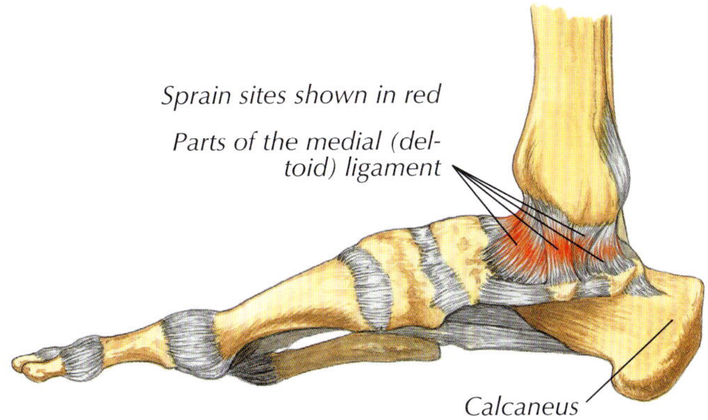

Description

Ankle sprain is either a grade one, two or three tear to one of the ankle ligaments and is the most common sports injury today; approximately 8.4 million in the USA and 1.5 million in the UK people seek medical treatment for ankle sprains each year. An inversion sprain is most common, which damages the lateral ligaments. The talofibular ligament is most commonly sprained ligament.

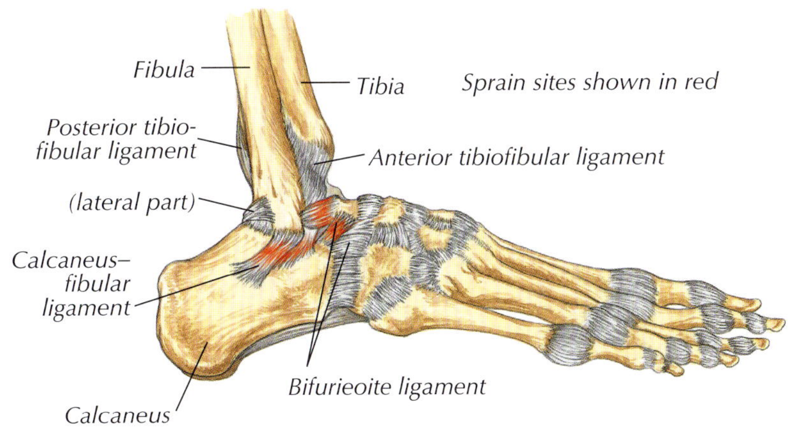

Symptoms

Grade 1

- Mild pain.
- May be mild swelling around the ankle.
- Some joint stiffness and difficulty walking or running.

Grade 2

- Moderate to severe pain.
- Swelling and stiffness, may be bruising.
- Some instability of the joint.
- Difficulty walking.

Grade 3

- Severe pain, usually followed by no pain.
- Extreme swelling, bruising and stiffness.
- Extreme instability of the joint.
- Unable to bear weight.

Causes

- Extreme inversion or eversion of the foot.
- Over pronation in the affected limb.
- Core instability (possible visceral inflammation)
- A lower cross syndrome.
- Impact injuries, such as car accidents or tackles in rugby or soccer when the foot is planted on the ground.

Treatment

Acute

- Always seek professional help if you suspect an ankle sprain. In the first 24 to 48 hours, use RICE to prevent further damage and optimize healing time.

Post-acute

- Mobilization of the ankle joint within pain-free ranges.
- Sports massage and corrective exercise.
- Strength training normally begins with isometric, then concentric and finally eccentric work is added.
- A total rupture usually requires surgery.

Exercises

Stretching

- Once the inflammation has ceased, the ankle should be gently moved into pain-free ranges of motion to recover the full range of motion of the joint and help re-align scar tissue.
- Any tight muscles around the hip, knee or ankle joints should be stretched within pain-free ranges. These will differ from person to person.

Strengthening

- Once weight-bearing is possible and inflammation has ceased, strengthen the following muscles: gluteus maximus, gluteus medius and minimus, transversus abdominus and external obliques.

RECOVERY TIME WITH APPROPRIATE RECOVERY MANAGEMENT
Grade 1 sprain: 2 to 3 weeks
Grade 2 sprain: 3 to 6 weeks
Grade 3 sprain: 3 to 6 months or more

See exercises

- *Calf stretch (page 107)*
- *Squat on balance board (page 124)*
- *Lunge (page 128)*

ANTERIOR COMPARTMENT SYNDROME

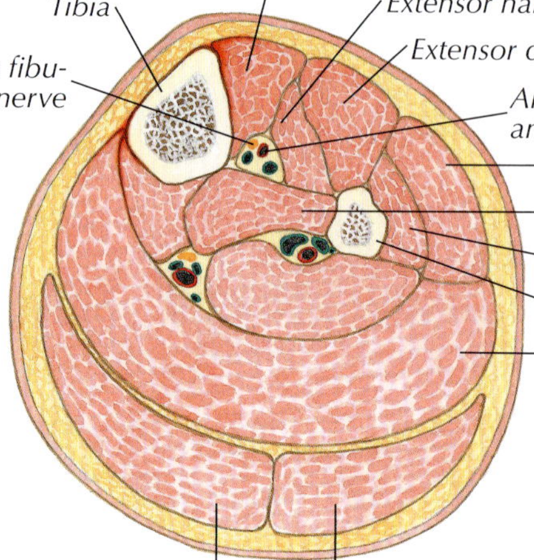

Description

This injury is the result of diffuse tightness and tenderness caused by an increase in pressure within the anterior compartment (tibialis anterior, extensor hallucis longus, extensor digitorum longus and peroneus brevis) within the surrounding fascia. The increase in pressure on the surrounding fascia is created when the muscles hypertrophy against the unyielding fascia and restrict circulation in the muscles.

Symptoms

- Swelling and tenderness over the tibialis anterior muscle, which does not respond to use of pain medication.
- Pain increases with exercise.
- Weakness with dorsiflexion of the ankle.
- Pain with dorsiflexion and plantar flexion of the ankle and flexion or extension of the toes.
- Tibialis anterior may feel hot to the touch and the area may be numb.
- Can lead to paralysis if not treated.

Causes

- Impact injury, muscle tear or over-use which can all lead to swelling.
- Over-pronation in the affected limb.
- Core instability (possible visceral inflammation).
- A lower cross syndrome.
- An aggressive increase in training intensity, duration, volume and/or frequency. A rapid increase in uphill running.

Treatment

Acute

- In the first 24 to 48 hours, use RICE to prevent further damage and optimize healing time.
- Anti-inflammatory protocols.

Post-acute

- Taping.
- Sports massage.
- Heat treatments.
- Corrective exercise, especially improving muscle balance in the lower limbs, leading to gradual return to training and competition.
- Strength training normally begins with isometric, then concentric and finally eccentric work is added.
- Surgery is sometimes used to release the pressure within the compartment.

RECOVERY TIME WITH APPROPRIATE RECOVERY MANAGEMENT
4 to 6 weeks

Exercises

Stretching

- Once the inflammation has ceased, the ankle plantar flexors and dorsi flexors should be gradually stretched to recover the full range of motion of the ankle joint
- Any tight muscles around the hip, knee or ankle joints should be stretched within pain-free ranges. These will differ from person to person.

Strengthening

- Once weight-bearing is possible and inflammation has ceased, gradually strengthen all the lower body muscles.

See exercises
- *Anterior tibialis (page 106)*

SHIN SPLINTS

Description

Generic pain of the anterior lower leg (shin) area is sometimes referred to as shin splints, but is also known as Medial Tibial Traction Periostitis (inflammation of the periostium of the tibial) or Medial Tibial Stress Syndrome. This injury is two to three times more common in females than males and is common amongst runners, tennis players and netball players and other sports requiring running, jumping and sprinting. Shin splints occur in 13 percent of runners.

Symptoms

- Pain over the medial lower half of the tibia.
- Pain often at the start of exercise, but eases during exercise.
- Pain often returns after exercise.
- There may be swelling and redness over the sight of pain.

Causes

- Traction forces on the periosteum from the muscles of the lower leg.
- Over-pronation in the affected limb.
- Core instability (possible visceral inflammation).
- A lower cross syndrome.
- Flat feet (functional or structural).
- A weakness of the anterior shin compared to the posterior shin.
- An aggressive increase in training intensity, duration, volume and/or frequency. A rapid increase in uphill running.
- Running on hard surfaces.
- Poor-fitting or old footwear.

Treatment

Acute

- Use RICE (see page 29) in the first 24 to 48 hours to prevent further damage and optimize healing time.
- Anti-inflammatory protocols.

Post-acute

- Taping.
- Sports massage.
- Corrective exercise, especially improving muscle balance in the lower limbs, leading to gradual return to training and competition. Stretching of the plantar flexors and strengthening of the dorsi flexors is required.
- Strength training normally begins with isometric, then concentric and finally eccentric work is added.
- Correct footwear.

Exercises

Stretching

- Once the inflammation has ceased, the ankle plantar flexors should be gradually stretched to recover the full range of motion of the joint.
- Any tight muscles around the hip, knee or ankle joints should be stretched within pain-free ranges. These will differ from person to person.

Strengthening

- Once weight-bearing is possible and inflammation has ceased, strengthen the following muscles: tibialis anterior, gluteus maximus, gluteus medius and minimus, transversus abdominus and external obliques.

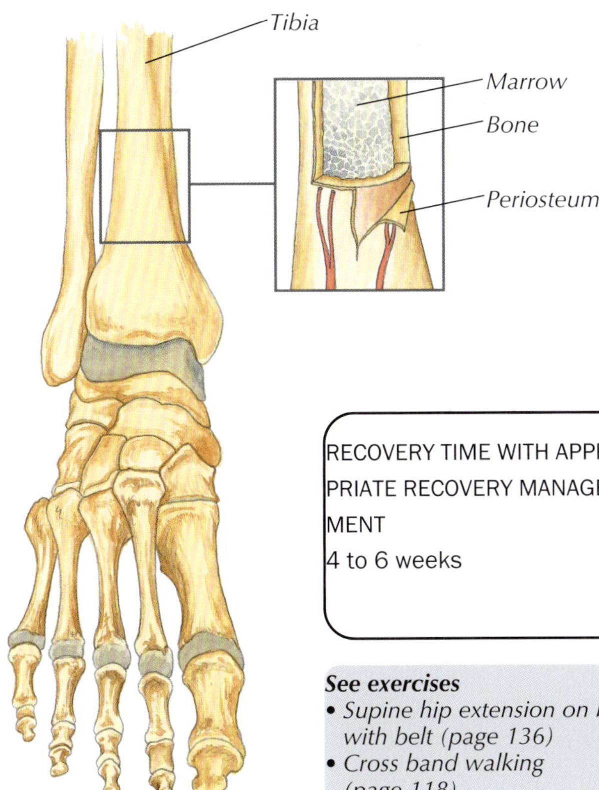

RECOVERY TIME WITH APPROPRIATE RECOVERY MANAGEMENT
4 to 6 weeks

See exercises
- *Supine hip extension on ball with belt (page 136)*
- *Cross band walking (page 118)*

KNEE INJURIES

ANTERIOR CRUCIATE LIGAMENT (ACL) SPRAIN

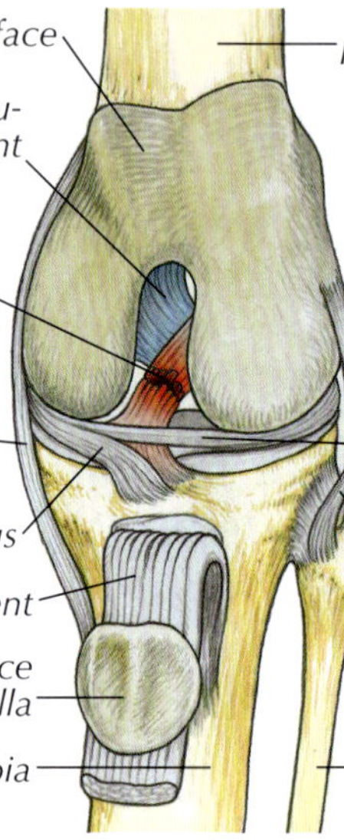

Description

The ACL resists anterior translation of the tibia in relation to the femur. Sprains are most common amongst 15–25 year olds who participate in sports that require a pivoting motion such as basketball, soccer and skiing. It is an injury more commonly suffered by women than by men. The medial collateral ligament and medial meniscus may be injured at the same time.

Symptoms

- Pain and instability, and swelling of the knee.
- Inability to bear weight on the affected knee.
- A loud pop may be heard if it is a complete tear.

Causes

- Often caused during a twisting motion of the knee when changing direction or pivoting.
- Over-pronation in the affected limb.
- Core instability (possible visceral inflammation).
- A lower cross syndrome.
- Impact injuries, such as car accidents or tackles in rugby or soccer when the foot is planted on the ground.

Treatment

Acute

- Use RICE in the first 24 to 48 hours to prevent further damage and optimize healing time.
- Seek professional help if you suspect an ACL sprain.
- Anti-inflammatory protocols.

Post-acute

- Sports massage and heat treatments.
- Corrective exercise, especially improving muscle balance in the lower limbs, leading to gradual return to training and competition.
- Strength training normally begins with isometric, then concentric and finally eccentric work is added.
- A total rupture usually requires surgery.

Exercises

Stretching

- Once the inflammation has ceased, the knee should be moved gently into pain-free ranges of motion to recover full range of motion of the joint and help re-align scar tissue
- Any tight muscles around the hip, knee or ankle joints should be stretched within pain-free ranges. These will differ from person to person.

Strengthening

- Once weight-bearing is possible and inflammation has ceased, strengthen gluteus maximus, medius and minimus, quadriceps, hamstrings, calves, transversus abdominus and external obliques.

RECOVERY TIME WITH APPROPRIATE RECOVERY MANAGEMENT
Grade 1 sprain: 2 to 3 weeks
Grade 2 sprain: 3 to 6 weeks
Grade 3 sprain: 3 to 6 months or more

See exercises
- *Four-point tummy vacuum (page 115)*
- *Squat on balance board (page 124)*
- *Lunge (page 128)*

BAKER'S CYST (POPLITEAL CYST)

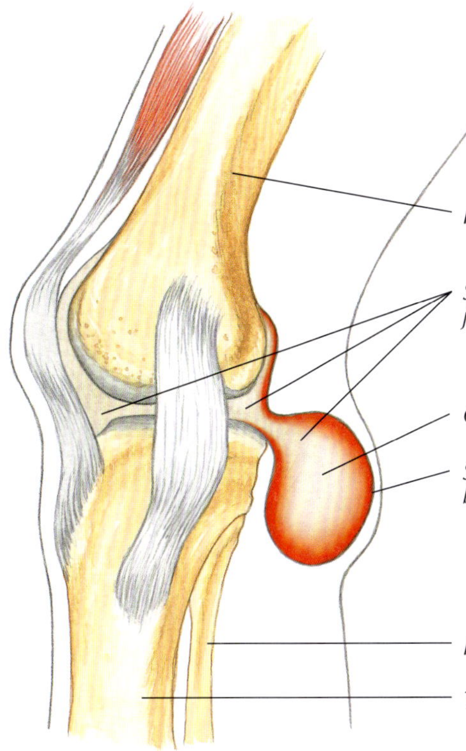

Description

Also known as Popliteal cyst, a baker's cyst is a swelling of the semimembranosus bursa caused by release of synovial fluid, just posterior to the medial condyle of the femur. It is a relatively rare condition.

Symptoms

- Swelling of the posterior knee and possibly calf muscles.
- Pain behind the knee and possibly in the calf muscles.
- Redness.
- May prevent bending of the knee and activity.

Causes

- Meniscal tear.
- Knee arthritis.
- Any knee injury.
- Has been associated with Lyme's disease.

Treatment

Acute

- Use RICE (see page 29) in the first 24 to 48 hours to prevent further damage and optimize healing time.
- Anti-inflammatory protocols.

Post-acute

- Sports massage.
- Corrective exercise, especially improving muscle balance in the lower limbs and lumbo-pelvic region, leading to gradual return to training (end-stage rehabilitation) and competition to prevent re-injury.
- Strength training normally begins with isometric, then concentric and finally eccentric work is added.
- In severe cases, surgical intervention is used to reduce swelling.

RECOVERY TIME WITH APPROPRIATE RECOVERY MANAGEMENT
2 to 12 weeks

Exercises

Stretching

- Once the inflammation has ceased, the knee should be gently moved into pain-free ranges of motion to recover the full range of motion of the joint and help re-align scar tissue.
- Any tight muscles around the pelvis, hip, knee or ankle joints should be gradually and progressively stretched within pain-free ranges. These muscles will differ from person to person.

Strengthening

- Once inflammation has ceased, strengthen the following muscles: gluteus maximus, gluteus medius and minimus, quadriceps, hamstrings, calves, transversus abdominus and external obliques.

See exercises
- *Four-point tummy vacuum (page 115)*
- *Squat on balance board (page 124)*
- *Lunge (page 128)*

CHONDROMALACIA PATELLA (RUNNER'S KNEE)

Description

Runner's knee is an irritation of the cartilage on the undersurface of the patella bone. The irritation is believed to occur when the patella rubs against one side of the knee joint during flexion of the knee, which causes pain at the front of the knee. It is common amongst young healthy athletes, especially cyclists, gymnasts, horse riders, rowers, runners, skateboarders, snowboarders, soccer players, tennis players and volleyball players. It is more common in females than males.

Symptoms

- Pain in the front of the knee around the kneecap.
- Pain may be deep-seated and radiate to the back of the knee.
- The pain may come and go, but is usually felt when squatting, kneeling, and going down stairs.

Causes

- Over-pronation in the affected limb.
- Core instability (possible visceral inflammation).
- A lower cross syndrome.
- A tight iliotibial band and patellar maltracking.
- Neuromas.
- Bursitis.
- Overuse.

Treatment

Acute

- Use RICE (see page 29) in the first 24 to 48 hours to prevent further damage and optimize healing time.
- Anti-inflammatory protocols.

Post-acute

- Sports massage.
- Heat treatments.
- Corrective exercise, especially improving muscle balance in the lower limbs, leading to gradual return to training and competition.
- Strength training normally begins with isometric, then concentric and finally eccentric work is added.

Exercises

Stretching

- The knee should be gently moved into pain-free ranges of motion to recover the full range of motion of the joint and help re-align scar tissue.
- Any tight muscles around the hip, knee or ankle joints should be stretched within pain-free ranges. These will differ from person to person.

Strengthening

- Strengthen the following muscles: gluteus maximus, gluteus medius and minimus, transversus abdominus and external obliques.

RECOVERY TIME WITH APPROPRIATE RECOVERY MANAGEMENT
3 to 8 weeks

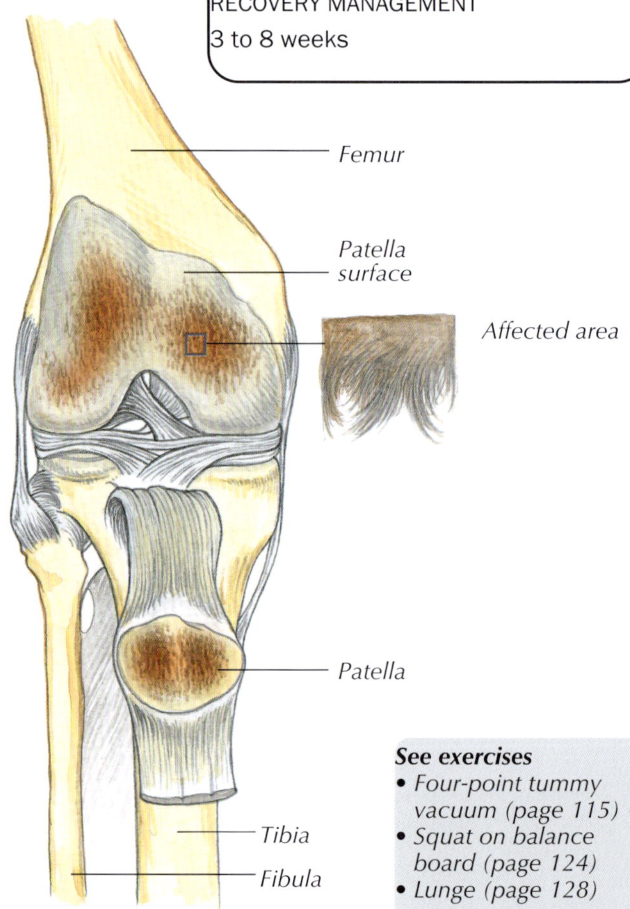

See exercises

- *Four-point tummy vacuum (page 115)*
- *Squat on balance board (page 124)*
- *Lunge (page 128)*

PATELLA TENDONITIS (JUMPER'S KNEE)

Description

Jumper's knee is an injury of the patella tendon (technically a ligament as it joins bone to bone) where it joins the patella. Micro-tears and collagen degeneration may occur in this injury. It is common amongst athletes that jump or change direction frequently, as in American football, basketball, bowling, golf, gymnastics, lacrosse, rugby and soccer, skateboarding, snowboarding, track and field, and volleyball.

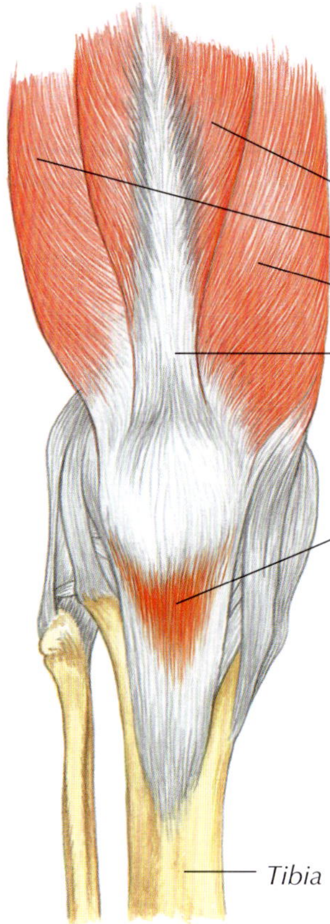

Symptoms

- Pain at the base of the patella.
- Pain to the touch.
- Pain with extension of the knee.
- May have a larger tendon on the affected side.

Causes

- Over-pronation in the affected limb.
- Core instability (possible visceral inflammation)
- A lower cross syndrome.
- Overuse (particularly jumping)

Treatment

Acute

- Use RICE (see page 29) in the first 24 to 48 hours to prevent further damage and optimize healing time.
- Anti-inflammatory protocols.

Post-acute

- Sports massage.
- Heat treatments.
- Corrective exercise, especially improving muscle balance in the lower limbs, leading to gradual return to training and competition.
- Strength training normally begins with isometric, then concentric and finally eccentric work is added.
- Surgery may be required in long-term cases.

RECOVERY TIME WITH APPROPRIATE RECOVERY MANAGEMENT
3 weeks to 3 months or more

Exercises

Stretching

- The knee should be gently moved into pain-free ranges of motion to recover the full range of motion of the joint and help re-align scar tissue.
- Any tight muscles around the hip, knee or ankle joints should be stretched within pain-free ranges. These will differ from person to person.

Strengthening

- Strengthen the following muscles: gluteus maximus, gluteus medius and minimus, gastrocnemius, quadriceps, transversus abdominus and external obliques.

See exercises
- *Four-point tummy vacuum (page 115)*
- *Squat on balance board (page 124)*
- *Lunge (page 128)*

MEDIAL CARTILAGE INJURY

Description

The meniscus is a crescent-shaped layer of cartilage that sits on top of the tibia. It provides shock absorption for the knee and weight transference between the tibia and femur. The medial meniscus is five times more susceptable to injury than the lateral meniscus due to its attachment to the medial collateral ligament and joint capsule. It can be injured along with the medial collateral ligament and the anterior cruciate ligament (the unhappy triad). This injury occurs in contact sports such as rugby and soccer when impacted (tackled) from the lateral side of the knee and during twisting and pivoting type movements such as basketball, skiing and tennis.

Symptoms

- Pain on the medial side of the knee.
- Swelling of the knee within the first 48 hours.
- Inability to bear weight on the affected knee.
- Pain with and inability to fully flex the knee.
- Popping or clicking within the knee.
- Locking or giving way of the knee.

Causes

- Often caused during a twisting motion of the knee when changing direction or pivoting.
- Over-pronation in the affected limb.
- Core instability (possible visceral inflammation).
- A lower cross syndrome.
- Impact to the lateral knee, such as tackles in rugby or soccer.

Knee joint seen from above

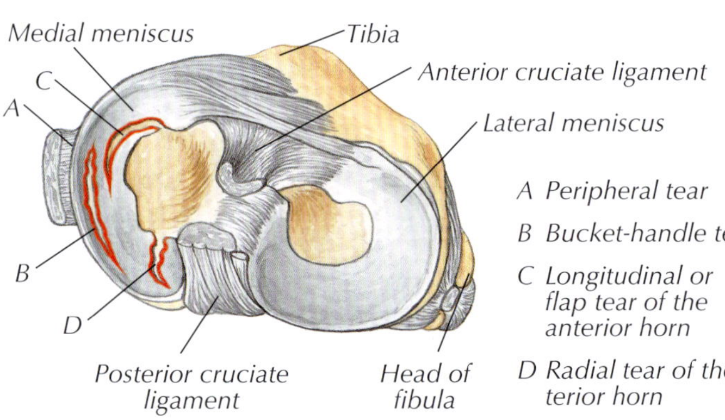

A Peripheral tear
B Bucket-handle tear
C Longitudinal or flap tear of the anterior horn
D Radial tear of the posterior horn

Treatment

Acute

- Use RICE (see page 29) in the first 24 to 48 hours to prevent further damage and optimize healing time.
- Anti-inflammatory protocols.

Post-acute

- Sports massage.
- Heat treatments.
- Corrective exercise, especially improving muscle balance in the lower limbs and lumbo-pelvic region, leading to gradual return to training and competition.
- Strength training normally begins with isometric, then concentric and finally eccentric work is added.
- Surgery may be required in some instances.

RECOVERY TIME WITH APPROPRIATE RECOVERY MANAGEMENT
2 weeks to 4 months or more

Exercises

Stretching

- Once the inflammation has ceased, the knee should be gently moved into pain-free ranges of motion to recover the full range of motion of the joint and help re-align scar tissue.
- Any tight muscles around the pelvis, hip, knee or ankle joints should be gradually and progressively stretched within pain-free ranges. These muscles will differ from person to person.

Strengthening

- Once weight bearing is possible and inflammation has ceased, strengthen the following muscles: gluteus maximus, gluteus medius and minimus, transversus abdominus and external obliques.

See exercises
- *Four-point tummy vacuum (page 115)*
- *Squat on balance board (page 124)*
- *Lunge (page 128)*

MEDIAL COLLATERAL LIGAMENT SPRAIN

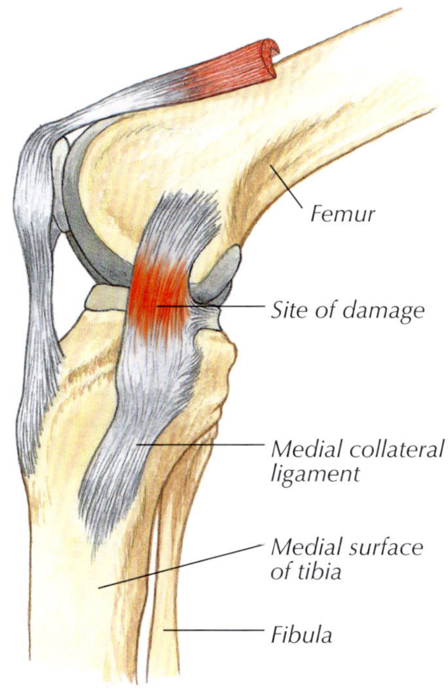

Description

The medial collateral ligament (MCL) is a broad, flat, membranous ligament that attaches from the medial condyle of the femur to just below the adductor tubercle of the tibia. Also known as the tibial collateral ligament, it provides stability to the knee by preventing the medial knee joint from adducting. MCL sprain is one of the most common knee ligament injuries and is prevalent amongst young athletes. It can be injured along with the medial cartilage and the anterior cruciate ligament (the unhappy triad). This injury occurs in contact sports such as American football, rugby and soccer when impacted (tackled) from the lateral side of the knee, and during twisting and pivoting movements such as those done in basketball, ice hockey, skiing and tennis.

Symptoms

- Pain over the ligament ranging from mild to severe.
- Swelling and bruising of the knee within the first 48 hours (grade 2 or 3).
- Joint laxity (grade 2 or 3).
- Locking or giving way of the knee.

Causes

- Often caused during a twisting motion of the knee when changing direction or pivoting.
- Over-pronation in the affected limb.
- Core instability (possible visceral inflammation).
- A lower cross syndrome.
- Impact to the lateral knee, such as tackles in American football, rugby or soccer.

Treatment

Acute

- Use RICE (see page 29) in the first 24 to 48 hours to prevent further damage and optimize healing time.
- Anti-inflammatory protocols.

Post-acute

- Knee support or cast may be required for grade 2 or 3.
- Sports massage.
- Heat treatments.
- Corrective exercise, especially improving muscle balance in the lower limbs and lumbo-pelvic region, leading to gradual return to training (end-stage rehabilitation) and competition.
- Strength training normally begins with isometric, then concentric and finally eccentric work is added.
- Surgery may be required for grade 3 tears.

RECOVERY TIME WITH APPROPRIATE RECOVERY MANAGEMENT
Grade 1 sprain: 2 to 3 weeks
Grade 2 sprain: 3 to 6 weeks
Grade 3 sprain: 3 to 4 months or more

Exercises

Stretching

- Once the inflammation has ceased, the knee should be moved gently into pain-free ranges of motion to recover the full range of motion of the joint and help re-align scar tissue.
- Any tight muscles around the pelvis, hip, knee or ankle joints should be gradually and progressively stretched within pain-free ranges. These muscles will differ from person to person.

Strengthening

- Once weight-bearing is possible and inflammation has ceased, strengthen the following muscles: gluteus maximus, gluteus medius and minimus, transversus abdominus and external obliques.

See exercises
- *Four-point tummy vacuum (page 115)*
- *Squat on balance board (page 124)*
- *Lunge (page 128)*

OSTEOARTHRITIS

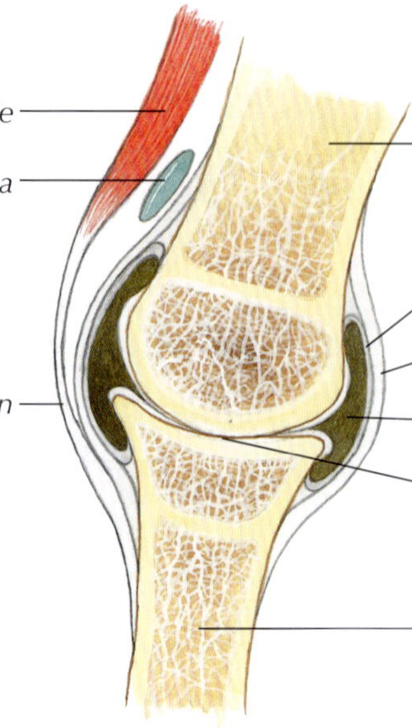

Description

Articular cartilage is a smooth fibrous layer of cartilage that covers the surfaces of bone; it allows smooth movement between bones and provides some shock absorption. Osteoarthritis (OA) is the inflammation and degeneration of that cartilage. Once the cartilage wears down it exposes rough bone, which creates more degeneration of the joint. The knee is the most common place for arthritis to occur. It is mostly seen in the older population, is more common in females and excess body weight is a risk factor. OA tends to occur in intense sports such as basketball, cricket, rugby and soccer.

Symptoms

- Pain.
- Swelling.
- Crepitus (grinding or crunching noise) during movement of the knee.
- Stiffness in the joint, particularly following a period of inactivity which tends to ease with movement.

Causes

- Overweight.
- Previous ligament or meniscus injury to the knee.
- Previous fracture to the joint.
- Over-use.
- Over-pronation in the affected limb.
- Core instability (possible visceral inflammation).

Treatment

Acute

- Use RICE (see page 29) in the first 24 to 48 hours to prevent further damage and minimize inflammation.
- Anti-inflammatory protocols

Post-acute

- Knee support or cast may be required.
- Sports massage.
- Heat treatments.
- Corrective exercise, especially improving muscle balance in the lower limbs and lumbo-pelvic region, leading to gradual return to training (end-stage rehabilitation) and competition.
- Strength training normally begins with isometric, then concentric and finally eccentric work is added.
- Surgery may be required.

RECOVERY TIME WITH APPROPRIATE RECOVERY MANAGEMENT
4 weeks to 6 months

Exercises

Stretching

- Once the inflammation has ceased, the knee should be moved gently into pain-free ranges of motion to recover the full range of motion of the joint and help re-align scar tissue.
- Any tight muscles around the pelvis, hip, knee or ankle joints should be gradually and progressively stretched within pain-free ranges. These muscles will differ from person to person.

Strengthening

- Once weight-bearing is possible and inflammation has ceased, strengthen the following muscles: gluteus maximus, gluteus medius and minimus, quadriceps, hamstrings, calves, transversus abdominus and external obliques.

See exercises

- *Four-point tummy vacuum (page 115)*
- *Squat on balance board (page 124)*
- *Lunge (page 128)*

POSTERIOR CRUCIATE LIGAMENT SPRAIN

Description

The Posterior cruciate ligament (PCL) connects the posterior intercondylar area of the tibia to the medial condyle of the femur. It resists posterior translation of the tibia, in relation to the femur. The PCL accounts for approximately 20 percent of all knee injuries; the lateral meniscus and articular cartilage can often be injured at the same time.

Symptoms

- Pain in the knee.
- Pain may also be felt in the calf region.
- Pain when the knee is extended under load.
- Limited range of motion.
- Possible swelling.
- Instability of the joint, often with the feeling of the knee giving way.

Causes

- Often trauma/impact to the front of the tibia when the knee is flexed forcing the shin backwards.
- A fall, landing on the knee joint while it is in full flexion.
- Shins hitting the dashboard of a car in a collision.

Treatment

Acute

- Use RICE (see page 29) in the first 24 to 48 hours to prevent further damage and optimize healing time.
- Anti-inflammatory protocols.

Post-acute

- Sports massage.
- Heat treatments.
- Corrective exercise.
- Strength training normally begins with isometric, then concentric and finally eccentric work is added.
- Surgery may be required in some cases.

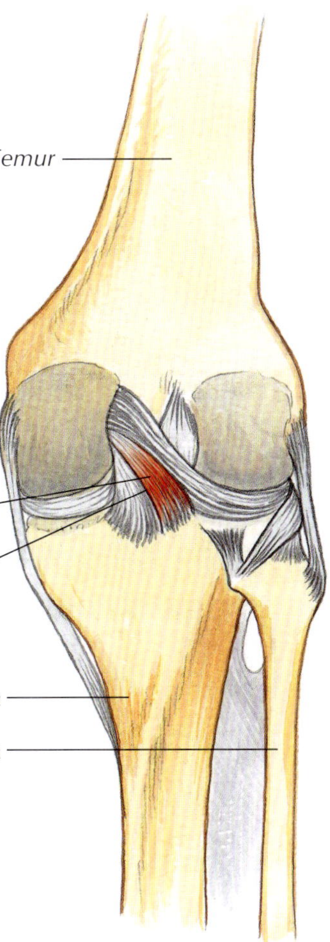

RECOVERY TIME WITH APPROPRIATE RECOVERY MANAGEMENT
Grade 1 sprain: 2 to 3 weeks
Grade 2 sprain: 3 to 6 weeks
Grade 3 sprain: 3 to 6 months or more

Exercises

Stretching

- The knee should be moved gently into pain-free ranges of motion to recover the full range of motion of the joint and help re-align scar tissue.
- Any tight muscles around the hip, knee or ankle joints should be stretched within pain-free ranges. These will differ from person to person.

Strengthening

- Strengthen the following muscles: gluteus maximus, gluteus medius and minimus, hamstrings group, gastrocnemius, quadriceps, transversus abdominus and external obliques.

See exercises
- *Lower abdominals (page 123)*
- *Squat on balance board (page 124)*
- *Romanian deadlift (page 131)*

QUADRICEPS TENDONITIS

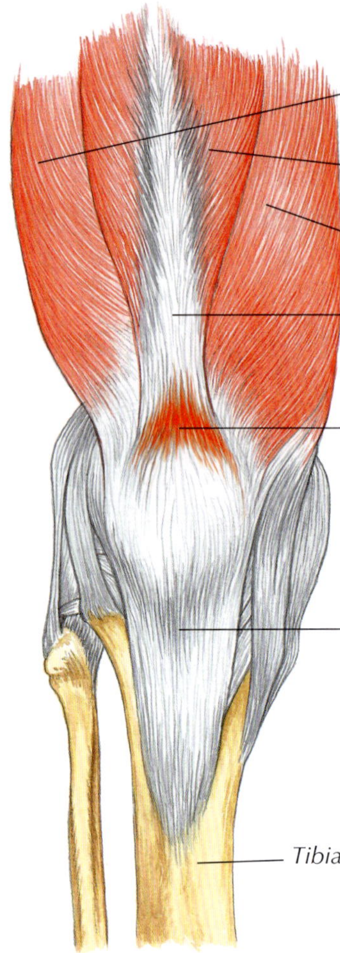

Description

The quadriceps tendon joins the quadriceps muscles to the patella. Quadriceps tendonitis is the inflammation of that tendon. This injury occurs most commonly to athletes who run, jump, stop and start quickly.

Symptoms

- Pain just above the patella.
- Swelling.
- Sensitive to touch.
- May prevent activity.

Causes

- Over-use.
- Premature return to training from a previous injury.
- Over-pronation in the affected limb.
- Core instability (possible visceral inflammation).

Treatment

Acute

- Use RICE (see page 29) in the first 24 to 48 hours to prevent further damage and optimize healing time.
- Anti-inflammatory protocols.

Post-acute

- Sports massage.
- Heat treatments.
- Corrective exercise, especially improving muscle balance in the lower limbs and lumbo-pelvic region, leading to gradual return to training (end-stage rehabilitation) and competition.
- Strength training normally begins with isometric, then concentric and finally eccentric work is added.

Exercises

Stretching

- Once the inflammation has ceased, the knee should be moved gently into pain-free ranges of motion to recover the full range of motion of the joint and help re-align scar tissue.
- Any tight muscles around the pelvis, hip, knee or ankle joints should be gradually and progressively stretched within pain-free ranges. These muscles will differ from person to person.

Strengthening

- Once weight bearing is possible and inflammation has ceased, strengthen the following muscles: gluteus maximus, gluteus medius and minimus, quadriceps, hamstrings, calves, transversus abdominus and external obliques.

RECOVERY TIME WITH APPROPRIATE RECOVERY MANAGEMENT
3 to 4 weeks

See exercises
- *Quadriceps stretch (page 111)*
- *Squat on balance board (page 124)*
- *Lunge (page 128)*

THIGH INJURIES

HAMSTRING ORIGIN TENDINOPATHY

Description

Damage or inflammation to the proximal hamstring tendon close to the ischial tuberosity (lower buttock) is a common injury in sports that require sprinting and fast acceleration, repetitive running, kicking and jumping. It is often considered an overuse injury.

Symptoms

- Pain, aching or stiffness around the ischial tuberosity.
- Pain with activity that may worsen after activity.
- Sensation of weakness in the affected limb, especially when trying to run.
- Pain stretching or contracting the hamstring muscles.

Causes

- Often occurs during sprinting as the hamstring muscles slow down the leg prior to heel-strike and are near full stretch.
- A forceful repetitive action, such as kicking, jumping or accelerating.
- One theory is a weak transversus abdominus muscle, therefore causing the biceps femoris to work harder to stabilize the sacroiliac joint.
- Another theory suggests a lengthened/weak gluteus maximus muscle causing the hamstrings to overwork to extend the hip (synergistic dominance).

Treatment

Acute

- Use RICE (see page 29) in the first 24 to 48 hours to prevent further damage and optimize healing time.
- Anti-inflammatory protocols.

Post-acute

- Sports massage.
- Corrective exercise, especially improving muscle balance in the lower limbs and lumbo-pelvic region, leading to gradual return to training (end-stage rehabilitation) and competition to prevent re-injury.
- Strength training normally begins with isometric, then concentric and finally eccentric work is added.

Exercises

Stretching

- Once the inflammation has ceased, the hip and knee should be moved gently into pain-free ranges of motion to recover the full range of motion of the joints and help re-align scar tissue.
- Any tight muscles around the pelvis, hip, knee or ankle joints should be gradually and progressively stretched within pain-free ranges. These muscles will differ from person to person.

Strengthening

- Once inflammation has ceased, strengthen the following muscles: gluteus maximus, hamstrings, transversus and abdominals.

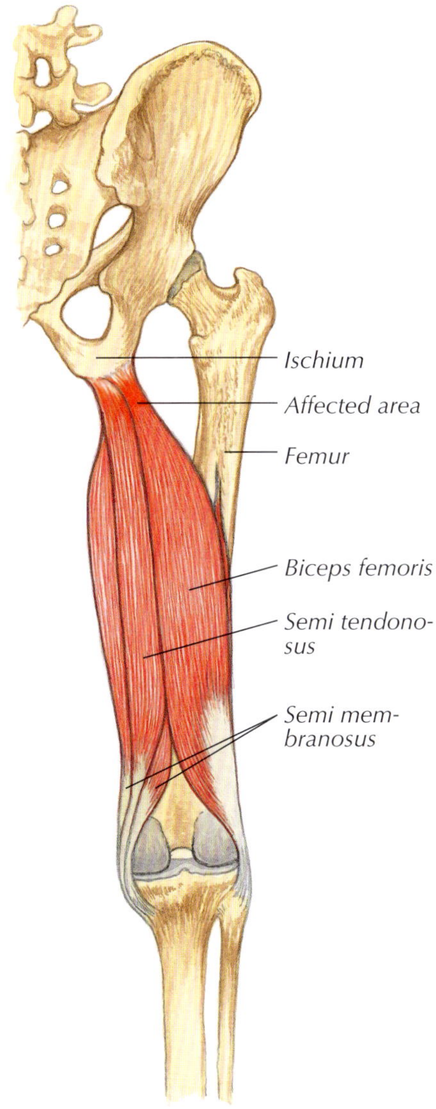

RECOVERY TIME WITH APPROPRIATE RECOVERY MANAGEMENT
3 to 6 weeks (if treated early enough)

See exercises

- *Four-point tummy vacuum (page 115)*
- *Supine hip extension on ball with belt (page 136)*
- *Lunge (page 128)*

HAMSTRING STRAIN

Description

Grades 1, 2 or 3 strains of one of the hamstring group muscles are common in sports that require sprinting and fast acceleration.

Symptoms

Grade 1

- Tightness/cramping sensation in the posterior thigh when the muscle is contracted or stretched.
- Some discomfort when walking.
- May be minimal swelling.

Grade 2

- Immediate severe pain is felt.
- Pain with stretching and contraction of the muscle.
- Gait will be affected; there may be limping.
- Swelling may be noticeable.
- May not be able to fully straighten the knee.

Grade 3

- Immediate severe pain and swelling.
- Constant pain.
- Gait will be severely affected and crutches are likely to be needed.

Causes

- Often occurs during sprinting as the hamstring muscles slow down the leg prior to heel-strike and are near full stretch.
- Lack of effective warm-up.
- One theory is a weak transversus abdominus muscle, therefore causing the biceps femoris to work harder to stabilize the sacroiliac joint.
- Another theory suggests a lengthened/weak gluteus maximus muscle causing the hamstrings to overwork to extend the hip (synergistic dominance).

Treatment

Acute

- Use RICE (see page 29) in the first 24 to 48 hours to prevent further damage and optimize healing time.
- Anti-inflammatory protocols.

Post-acute

- Sports massage.
- Corrective exercise, especially improving muscle balance in the lower limbs and lumbo-pelvic region, leading to gradual return to training (end-stage rehab) and competition to prevent re-injury.
- Strength training normally begins with isometric, then concentric and finally eccentric work is added.
- For grade 3 tears, surgery may be required.

Exercises

Stretching

- Once the inflammation has ceased, the hip and knee should be moved gently into pain-free ranges of motion to recover the full range of motion of the joint and help re-align scar tissue.
- Any tight muscles around the pelvis, hip, knee or ankle joints should be gradually and progressively stretched within pain-free ranges. These muscles will differ from person to person.

Strengthening

- Once inflammation has ceased, strengthen the following muscles: gluteus maximus, hamstrings, transversus and abdominals.

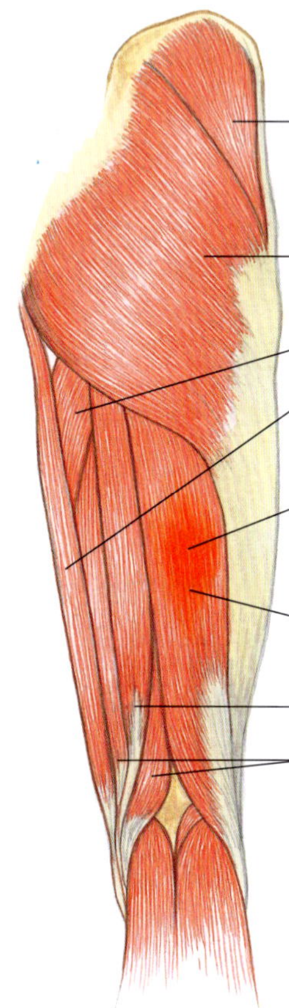

RECOVERY TIME WITH APPROPRIATE RECOVERY MANAGEMENT
Grade 1 strain: Days
Grade 2 strain: 3 to 6 weeks
Grade 3 strain: 2 to 3 months

See exercises

- *Four-point tummy vacuum (page 115)*
- *Romanian deadlift (page 131)*
- *Lunge (page 128)*

MYOSITIS OSSIFICANS

Description

This injury is a non-hereditary painful condition where damaged muscle tissue calcifies (becomes bone) following trauma. It most commonly occurs in the quadriceps muscles and bone growth begins within two to four weeks and matures after three to six months. 'Myositis ossificans progressiva' is a genetic condition where bone calcifies without trauma, but is very rare.

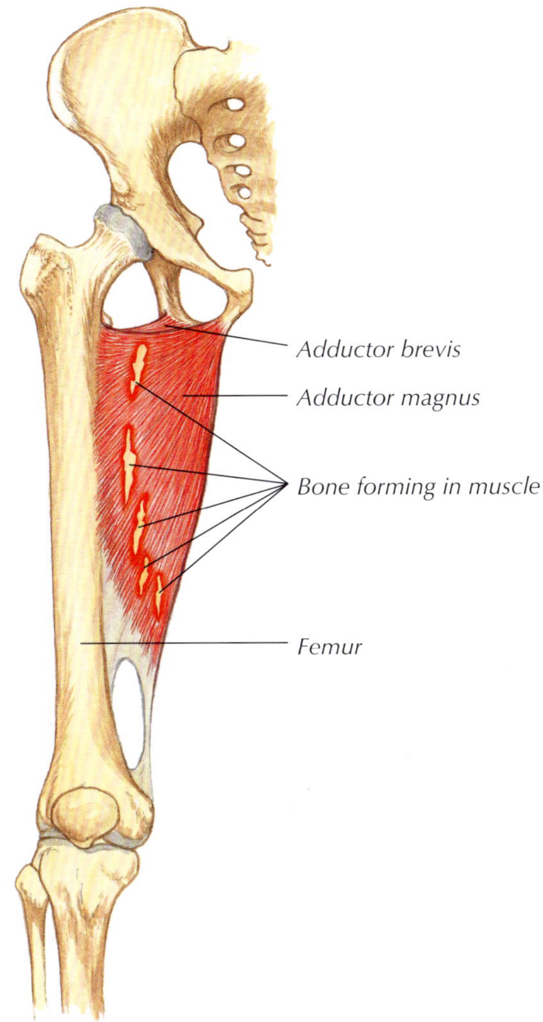

Symptoms

- Pain.
- Hardness in the muscle.
- Restricted range of motion.

Causes

- A collision injury where there is damage to the muscle and the periostium (fascial sheath surrounding the bone).
- Not applying RICE straight after the intial injury.
- Premature aggressive manual therapy (massage techniques).
- A premature return to training and/or competition.

Treatment

- An X-ray should be used to confirm the condition.
- Rest the affected limb.
- Inflammatory protocols.
- In some cases, surgery can be required after six months if affecting movement or irritating a nerve.

Exercises

No specific stretching or strengthening exercises.

RECOVERY TIME WITH APPROPRIATE RECOVERY MANAGEMENT
3 to 4 weeks

QUADRICEPS CONTUSION (DEAD-LEG)

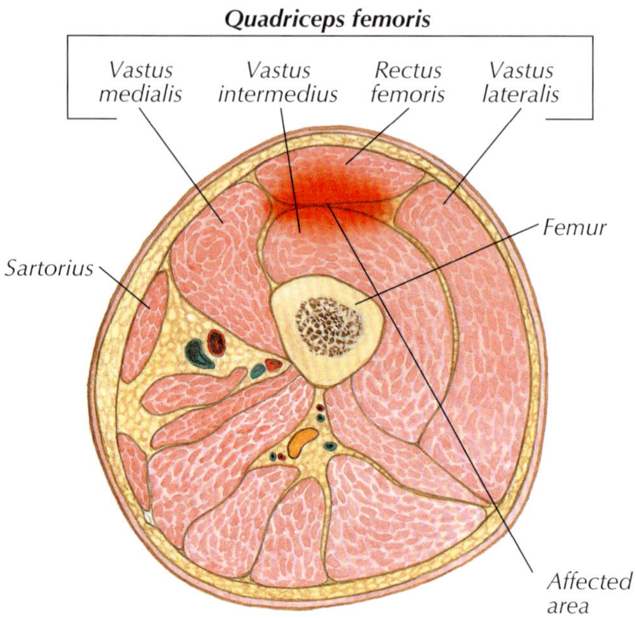

Description

This injury is caused by bruising to the skin, muscles, fascia or bone in the front of the thigh normally due to a collision. It is common in sports that involve contact with the thigh, including rugby, American football and soccer. Bleeding can be intramuscular (within the fascial sheath) or intermuscular (through the fascial sheath into surrounding tissues).

Symptoms

- Pain, tenderness and swelling in the anterior thigh.
- Redness, progressing to the black, blue and purple bruising colour.

Causes

- A collision injury where one or more of the quadriceps muscles is crushed against the femur.

Treatment

Acute

- Use RICE (see page 29) in the first 24 to 48 hours to prevent further damage and optimize healing time.
- Anti-inflammatory protocols.

Post-acute

- Sports massage.
- In rare instances, surgery may be required to remove blood clots.

RECOVERY TIME WITH APPROPRIATE RECOVERY MANAGEMENT
3 days to 12 weeks

Exercises

Stretching

- Once the inflammation has ceased, the hip and knee should be moved gently into pain-free ranges of motion to recover the full range of motion of the joints and help realign scar tissue.

Strengthening

- Upper body training can continue as long as standing is pain free.
- Once inflammation has ceased, a gradual return to normal training should commence.

QUADRICEPS STRAIN

Description

A grade 1, 2 or 3 strain of one of the quadriceps group muscles, this injury is common in sports that require running, kicking and jumping. The most common quadriceps muscle strained is the rectus femoris and the most common site of strain is the musculotendinous junction just above the knee.

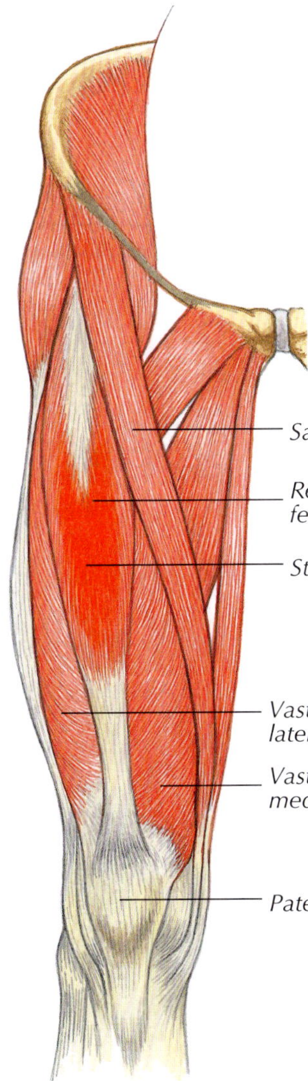

Symptoms

Grade 1

- Twinge, tightness and mild discomfort.
- May have discomfort with walking.
- Little to no swelling.
- Possible muscle spasm around the tear.

Grade 2

- Mild to severe pain in the area of the tear.
- Pain with walking or climbing stairs.
- Inability to continue activities/sport.
- Swelling.
- Bruising.
- Inability to fully flex or extend knee.

Grade 3

- Severe pain in the thigh.
- Inability to walk.
- Rapid swelling.
- Bruising after 24 hours.
- Visible deformity may be seen in the muscle.

Causes

- Forceful action of kicking, jumping or sprinting.

Treatment

Acute

- Use RICE (see page 29) in the first 24 to 48 hours to prevent further damage and optimize healing time.
- Anti-inflammatory protocols.

Post-acute

- Sports massage.
- Corrective exercise, especially improving muscle balance in the lower limbs and lumbo-pelvic region, leading to gradual return to training (end-stage rehab) and competition to prevent re-injury.
- Strength training normally begins with isometric, then concentric and finally eccentric work is added.

RECOVERY TIME WITH APPROPRIATE RECOVERY MANAGEMENT
Grade 1 sprain: Days
Grade 2 sprain: 3 to 6 weeks
Grade 3 sprain: 2 to 3 months

Exercises

Stretching

- Once the inflammation has ceased, the hip and knee should be moved gently into pain-free ranges of motion to recover the full range of motion of the joints and help re-align scar tissue.
- Any tight muscles around the pelvis, hip, knee or ankle joints should be gradually and progressively stretched within pain-free ranges. These muscles will differ from person to person.

Strengthening

- Once inflammation has ceased, strengthen the following muscles: quadriceps, gluteus maximus, hamstrings, and transversus abdominus.

See exercises
- *Four-point tummy vacuum (page 115)*
- *Supine hip extension on ball with belt (page 136)*
- *Lunge (page 128)*

STRESS FRACTURE OF THE FEMUR

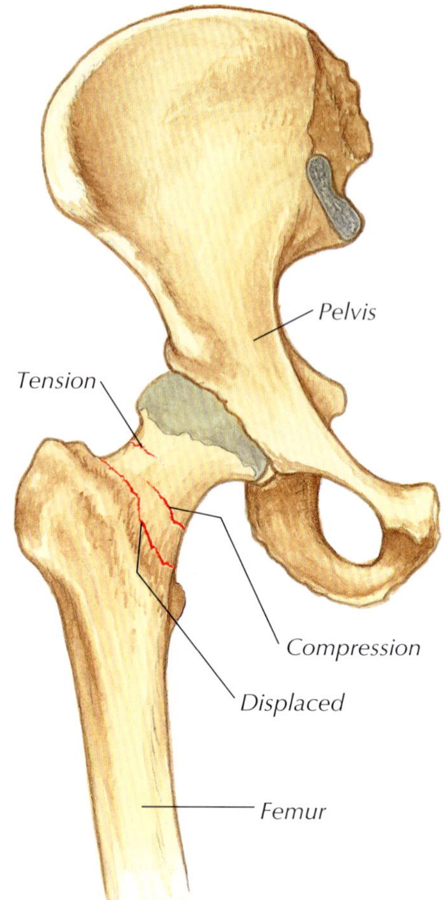

Description

Fracture to the femur due to overuse is an injury more likely to occur in endurance athletes, such as marathon and ultra-distance runners and Ironman triathletes. Insufficiency fractures occur when the training volume is not excessive, but there is insufficiency in the bone to take normal loads.

Symptoms

- Dull ache in the region of the fracture, which may be felt in the knee or hip joints depending on its specific location.
- Pain with weight-bearing.
- Inability to continue normal activity.

Causes

- A too-aggressive increase in training volume.
- Over-pronation.
- A problem with normal bone development.

Treatment

Acute

- An MRI and/or X-ray should be used to confirm the condition.
- Rest the affected limb.
- Inflammatory protocols.

Post-acute

- Following X-ray confirming no fracture, corrective exercise, especially improving muscle balance in the lower limbs and lumbo-pelvic region, leading to gradual return to training (end-stage rehab) and competition.
- Strength training normally begins with isometric, then concentric and finally eccentric work is added.

Exercises

Stretching

- When possible, the knee and hip should be moved gently into pain-free ranges of motion to recover the full range of motion of the joints.
- Any tight muscles around the pelvis, hip, knee or ankle joints should be gradually and progressively stretched within pain-free ranges. These muscles will differ from person to person.

Strengthening

- Water jogging should be used initially to allow gait with less stress on the bone.
- Once the X-ray shows a regrowth of bone and weight bearing is bearable, strengthen the following muscles: gluteus maximus, gluteus medius and minimus, transversus abdominus and external obliques.

RECOVERY TIME WITH APPROPRIATE RECOVERY MANAGEMENT
6 to 12 weeks

See exercises
- *Water jogging (page 137)*
- *Supine hip extension on ball with belt (page 136)*
- *Lunge (page 128)*

GROIN INJURIES

GILMORE'S GROIN

Description

Gilmore's groin is a torn external oblique aponeurosis, a dilation of the superficial inguinal ring, a torn conjoined tendon detached from the pubic tubercle and a separation of the conjoined tendon from the inguinal ligament. There is no herniation with Gilmore's groin. Typical sufferers are male adults participating in kicking sports and/or multi-directional sports that require rapid twisting and turning movements.

Symptoms

- Groin pain and weakness during sport.
- Pain may radiate into the adductor muscles and possibly the testes.
- Groin stiffness and soreness following sport.
- Inability to sprint, turn, twist or kick without discomfort and/or a lack of speed.
- Coughing, sneezing or laughing may produce pain.

Causes

- Believed to be caused by trauma or by over-use of sprinting, kicking, twisting and changing direction.
- Lack of effective warm-up.
- Inability to stabilize the pelvis during ballistic movement (weak core).
- Tight adductor muscles.
- Genetic factors.

Treatment

- Requires surgery, followed by all stages of normal rehabilitation through to end-stage rehabilitation.

RECOVERY TIME WITH APPROPRIATE RECOVERY MANAGEMENT
6 to 12 weeks following surgery

Exercises

Stretching

- Once the inflammation has ceased, the hip and knee should be moved gently into pain-free ranges of motion to recover the full range of motion of the joint and help realign scar tissue.
- Any tight muscles around the pelvis, hip, knee or ankle joints should be gradually and progressively stretched within pain-free ranges. These muscles will differ from person to person.

Strengthening

- Once inflammation has ceased, strengthen the following muscles: gluteus maximus, medius and minimus, quadriceps, hamstrings, abdominals, quadratus lumborum, latissimus dorsi.

See exercises
- *Lower abdominals (page 123)*
- *Supine lateral ball roll (page 125)*
- *Single-arm cable push (page 132)*

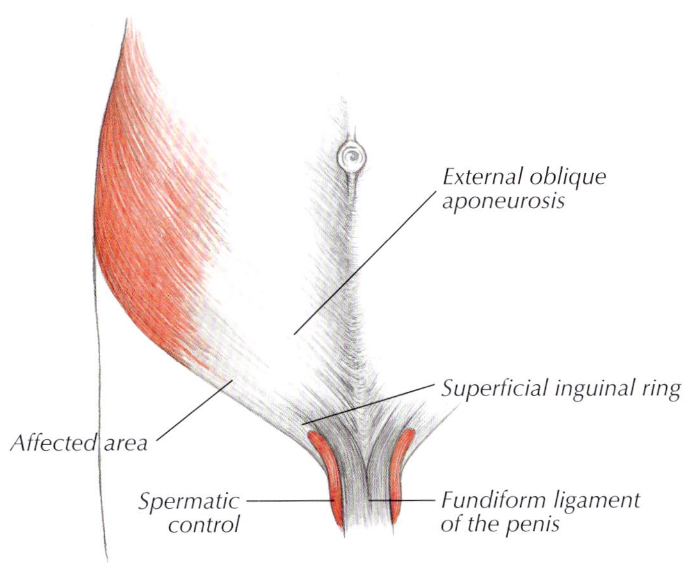

GROIN STRAIN

Description

A grade 1, 2 or 3 strain of one of the adductor muscles, groin strain injuries are common in sports that require sprinting, fast changes in direction and kicking. Soccer, rugby, tennis, ice hockey, American football and sprinting are sports particularly vulnerable to groin strains. Total ruptures are rare.

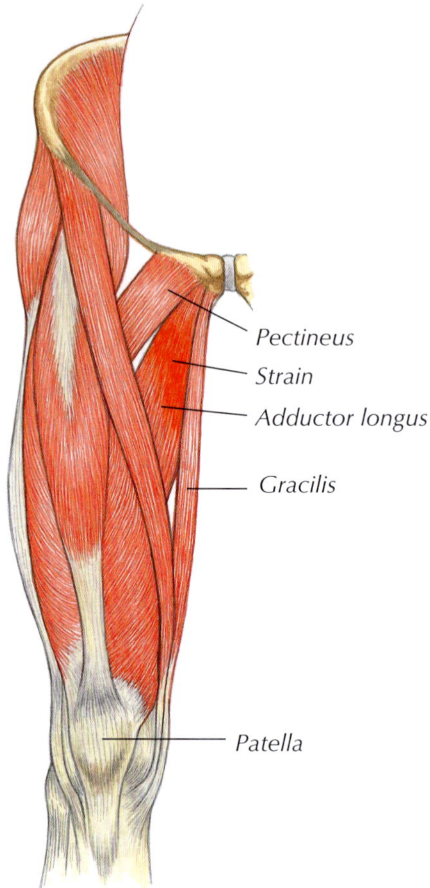

Symptoms

Grade 1

- Some discomfort may be present when walking.
- Activity may still be possible.
- Discomfort worse after activity.
- Muscular tightness.
- May be minimal swelling.

Grade 2

- Moderate to severe pain.
- Pain with stretching and contraction of the muscle.
- Pain with a change in direction.
- Muscular tightness.
- Gait affected; limping possible.
- Swelling and bruising may be noticeable.

Grade 3

- Immediate severe pain during sprinting or change of direction.
- Muscular spasm.
- Severe swelling and bruising (often after 24 hours.)
- Gait will be severely affected.

Causes

- Repetitive micro-trauma to the muscles caused by the lengthening and contracting of the muscles during running and kicking.
- Repetitive micro-trauma to the muscles caused by deceleration and acceleration during fast changes of direction.
- Lack of effective warm-up.
- Inability to stabilize pelvis during ballistic movement (weak core).
- Tight or weak adductor muscles.

Treatment

Acute

- Use RICE (see page 29) in the first 24 to 48 hours to prevent further damage and optimize healing time.
- Anti-inflammatory protocols.

Post-acute

- Sports massage.
- Corrective exercise, especially improving muscle balance in the lower limbs and lumbo-pelvic region, leading to gradual return to training (end-stage rehab) and competition to prevent re-injury.
- Strength training normally begins with isometric, then concentric and finally eccentric work is added.
- For grade 3 tears, surgery may be required.

RECOVERY TIME WITH APPROPRIATE RECOVERY MANAGEMENT
Grade 1 strain: Days
Grade 2 strain: 3 to 6 weeks
Grade 3 strain: 2 to 3 months

Exercises

Stretching

- Once the inflammation has ceased, the hip and knee should be moved gently into pain-free ranges of motion to recover the full range of motion of the joint and help re-align scar tissue.
- Any tight muscles around the pelvis, hip, knee or ankle joints should be gradually and progressively stretched within pain-free ranges. These muscles will differ from person to person.

Strengthening

- Once inflammation has ceased, strengthen the following muscles: gluteus maximus, medius and minimus, quadriceps, hamstrings, abdominals, quadratus lumborum, latissimus dorsi.

See exercises
- *Adductors (page 105)*
- *Supine hip extension on ball with belt (page 136)*

INGUINAL HERNIA

Description

An inguinal hernia is a protrusion of viscera through the abdominal wall through a gap in the inguinal canal. Direct hernias occur when abdominal contents protrude through a weakening in the abdominal wall into the inguinal canal. Indirect hernias occur when part of the abdomen bulges through the deep inguinal ring due to a birth defect and is less common. Inguinal hernia sufferers are typically male adults, participating in kicking sports and/or multi- directional sports that require rapid twisting and turning movements. Soccer, rugby, American football and sprinting are some sports that have a higher risk of inguinal hernia.

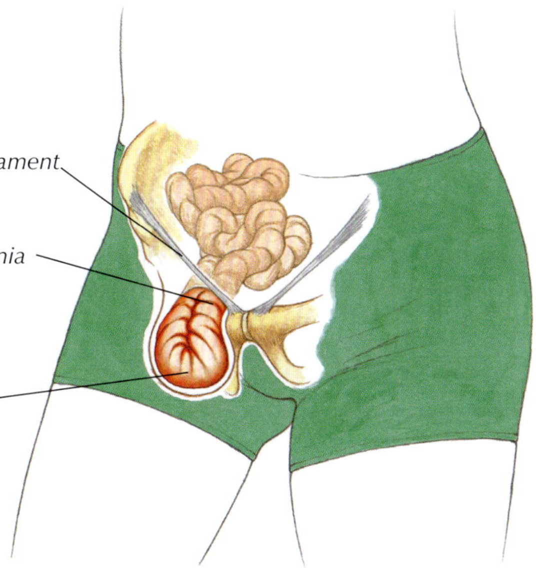

Symptoms

Non-traumatic

- A bulge in the groin that disappears when you lie down.
- Dull intermittent 'toothache'-like pain.
- Pain rarely radiates into the adductor muscles.
- Pain increases as exercise intensity increases, then subsides as fatigue sets in.
- Coughing, sneezing or laughing may produce pain.

Traumatic

- A solid swelling in the groin/lower abdominal/genital area following trauma, i.e. a rugby tackle.
- Constant pain.
- Sharp pain, swelling and discolouration in the area.

Causes

- Trauma or by over-use of sprinting, kicking, twisting and changing direction.
- Inability to stabilize the pelvis during ballistic movement (weak core).
- Weak abdominal muscles.
- Genetic factors.

Treatment

- Requires surgery, followed by all stages of normal rehabilitation to end-stage rehabilitation.

RECOVERY TIME WITH APPROPRIATE RECOVERY MANAGEMENT
6 to 8 weeks following surgery

Exercises

Stretching

- Once the inflammation has ceased, the hip and knee should be moved gently into pain-free ranges of motion to recover the full range of motion of the joint and help re-align scar tissue.
- Any tight muscles around the pelvis, hip, knee or ankle joints should be gradually and progressively stretched within pain-free ranges. These muscles will differ from person to person.

Strengthening

- Once inflammation has ceased, strengthen the following muscles: transversus abdominus, internal obliques and external obliques.

See exercises
- *Four-point tummy vacuum (page 115)*
- *Lower abdominals (page 123)*
- *Wood chop (page 138)*

OSTEITIS PUBIS

Description

A rare condition where there is inflammation of the pubic symphasis. It occurs mostly in soccer, hockey and American football players. The diagnosis is often confused with a groin strain.

Symptoms

- Pain in the region of the lower abdomen/pubic bone/pubic symphysis region.
- Pain can be more to one side.
- Possible limping.
- Weakness may also be felt in the affected limb.

Causes

- It usually develops following chronic repetitive movement of the symphysis pubis such as sprinting, kicking and twisting, which produces shearing and tensile forces and subsequent laxity in the symphysis ligament.
- Inability to stabilize the pelvis during ballistic movement (weak core).
- Overtraining.
- Leg-length discrepancy.

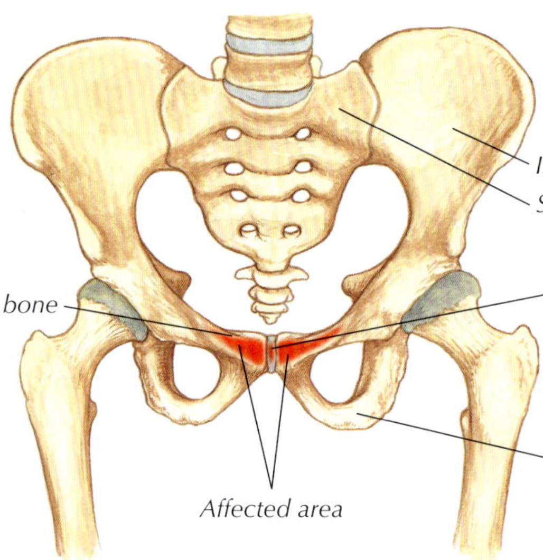

Treatment

Acute

- Initial rest and icing of the area.
- Anti-inflammatory protocols.

Post-acute

- Atlas re-alignment by a NUCCA chiropractor and a corrective exercise programme to overcome functional leg length discrepancy (common).
- Orthotics to help a structural leg-length discrepancy (very rare).

RECOVERY TIME WITH APPROPRIATE RECOVERY MANAGEMENT
Can take several months

Exercises

Stretching

- Any tight muscles around the pelvis, hip, knee or ankle joints should be gradually and progressively stretched within pain-free ranges. These muscles will differ from person to person.

Strengthening

- Strengthen any weak or long muscles around the lumbo-pelvic-hip region, abdominal or lower limbs based on the results of a biomechanical assessment.

GLUTEAL INJURIES

HIP BURSITIS

RECOVERY TIME WITH APPROPRIATE RECOVERY MANAGEMENT
1 to 4 weeks

Description

A painful condition caused by inflammation of one of the bursa in the hip region, hip bursitis occurs mostly in sports that require running, such as soccer, American football and long-distance running. When the bursa is inflamed the iliotibial band will rub against it with every stride causing further irritation. It can also be caused by an impact injury, such as falling onto hard ground and landing on the hip, e.g. a goalkeeper in soccer.

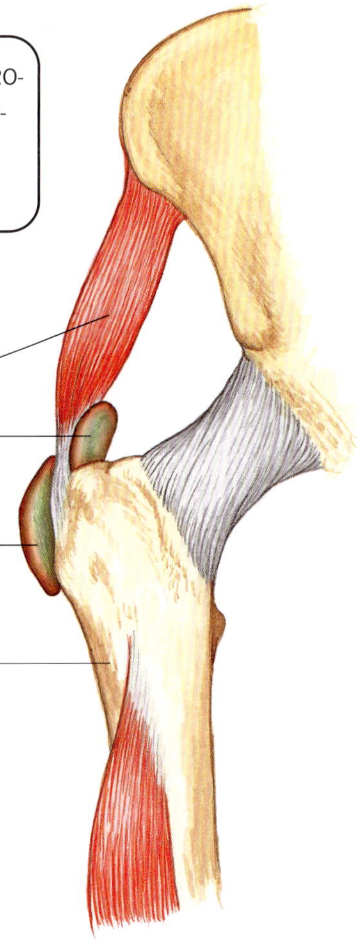

Symptoms

- Pain, tenderness and swelling over the lateral hip.
- Pain may radiate down the leg.
- Pain worsens with walking, running or climbing stairs.

Causes:

- Poor muscle balance/posture.
- Over-use.
- Over-pronation in the affected limb.
- Leg length discrepancy.
- Core instability (possible visceral inflammation).
- A hard fall onto the affected hip.

Treatment

Acute

- Use RICE (see page 29) in the first 24 to 48 hours to prevent further damage and optimize healing time.
- Anti-inflammatory protocols.

Post-acute

- Sports massage.
- Heat treatments.
- Corrective exercise, especially improving muscle balance in the lower limbs and lumbo-pelvic region, leading to gradual return to training (end-stage rehab) and competition.
- Strength training normally begins with isometric, then concentric and finally eccentric work is added.

Exercises

Stretching

- The tensor fascia lata muscle may need particular attention to prevent rubbing by the iliotibial band.
- Any tight muscles around the pelvis, hip, knee or ankle joints should be gradually and progressively stretched within pain-free ranges. These muscles will differ from person to person.

Strengthening

- Once weight bearing is possible and inflammation has ceased, strengthen the following muscles: gluteus maximus, gluteus medius and minimus, quadriceps, hamstrings, calves, transversus abdominus and external obliques.

See exercises
- *Tensor fascia lata (page 112)*
- *Cross band walking (page 118)*
- *Touch toe drill (page 126)*

PIRIFORMIS SYNDROME

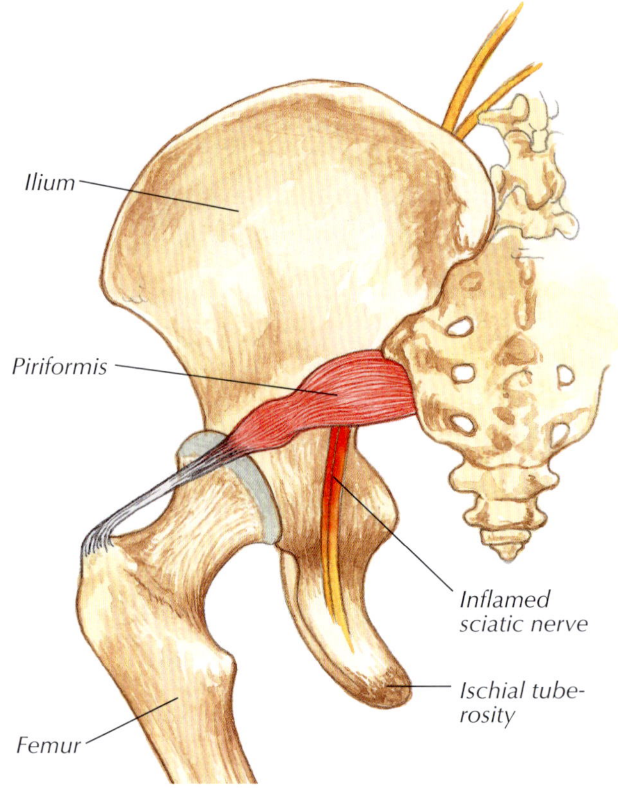

Description

The piriformis is a small muscle that originates on the lateral anterior surface of the sacrum and inserts onto the greater trochanter of the femur. The piriformis muscle rotates the hip externally and helps to stabilize the hip and sacroiliac joints. Piriformis syndrome is a painful condition in the buttock and posterior thigh region caused by irritation of the sciatic nerve by the piriformis muscle. It can be confused with similar symptoms caused by a disc bulge in the lumbar spine or confused with hamstring strain and hamstring tendinopathy. Seated sports such as rowing and cycling are particularly vulnerable.

Symptoms

- Pain, tingling, aching pain or numbness in the buttock.
- Pain may radiate down the leg all the way down to the hamstrings, calf and sometimes into the foot.

Causes

- Tightening, spasm or scar tissue of the piriformis muscle.
- Hematoma in the piriformis following trauma.
- Core instability.
- Over-pronation of the affected leg.
- Sacroiliac joint instability.
- Weak hip abductors and tight hip adductor muscles.
- A hard fall (trauma) to the affected piriformis muscle.

Treatment

Acute

- Rest and ice.
- Anti-inflammatory protocols.
- Neuromuscular Therapy™.
- Active Release Technique®.

Post-acute

- Heat treatments, contrast cold and hot.
- Stretching of the piriformis muscle (not all cases).
- Corrective exercise, especially improving muscle balance in the lower limbs and lumbo-pelvic region, leading to gradual return to training (end-stage rehab) and competition.
- Surgery in extreme cases.

RECOVERY TIME WITH APPROPRIATE RECOVERY MANAGEMENT
6 to 8 weeks
Up to 3 months after surgery

Exercises

Stretching

- The piriformis and adductor muscles may need particular attention to prevent the irritation on the sciatic nerve.
- Any tight muscles around the pelvis, hip, knee or ankle joints should be gradually and progressively stretched within pain-free ranges. These muscles will differ from person to person.

Strengthening

- Once weight bearing is possible and inflammation has ceased, strengthen the following muscles: gluteus maximus, gluteus medius and minimus, transversus abdominus and external obliques.

See exercises
- *Four-point tummy vacuum (page 115)*
- *Supine lateral ball roll (page 125)*
- *Cross band walking (page 118)*

SACROILIAC JOINT DYS-FUNCTION

Description

The sacroiliac joint (SIJ) is an L-shaped joint in between the ilium and sacrum. SIJ dysfunction is a painful condition caused by inflammation of one of the SIJs and is a common cause of back pain.

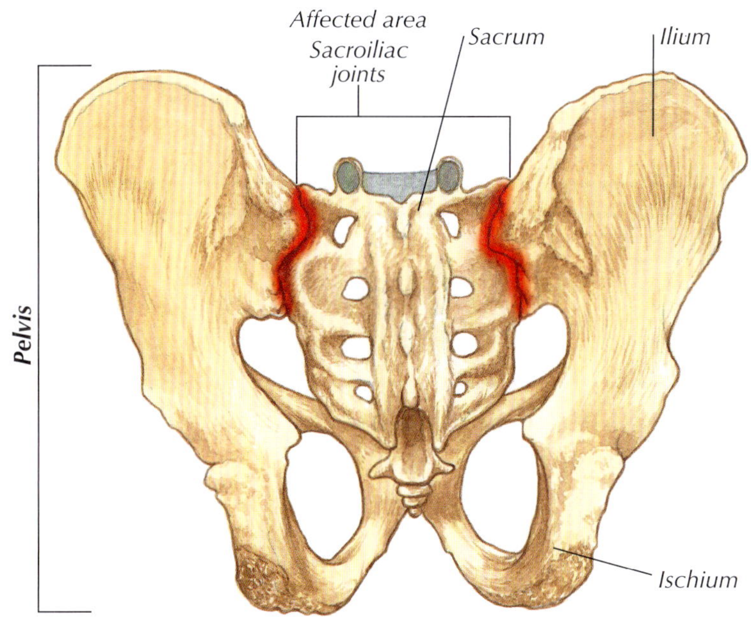

Symptoms

- A mild to moderate dull ache in the lower back around the posterior superior iliac spine (PSIS).
- Normally on one side, but can be on both.
- Pain can become worse or sharp during activity.
- Pain can refer to the hip, buttocks, groin and posterior thigh.
- May have muscle spasm in the gluteal muscles.

Causes

- Muscle imbalance around the lumbo-pelvic region.
- Core instability.
- Atlas (C1) subluxation (see page 73).
- Leg length discrepancy – functional (common) or structural (very rare).
- Arthritic conditions.
- Trauma, such as a car accident.
- Pregnancy.

Treatment

- Rest from normal sporting activities.
- Anti-inflammatory protocols.
- Sports massage and/or Neuromuscular Therapy™.
- SIJ manipulation (physiotherapy).
- Atlas re-alignment (NUCCA chiropractic).
- Corrective exercise, especially improving muscle balance in the lower limbs and lumbo-pelvic region, leading to gradual return to training (end-stage rehab) and competition.

RECOVERY TIME WITH APPROPRIATE RECOVERY MANAGEMENT
3 to 6 weeks

Exercises

Stretching

- Any tight muscles around the pelvis, hip, knee or ankle joints should be gradually and progressively stretched within pain-free ranges. These muscles will differ from person to person.

Strengthening

- Strengthen any weak muscles around the lumbo-pelvic region. These muscles will differ from person to person, but commonly include the transversus abdominus, multifidus, gluteus maximus, latissimus dorsi, erector spinae, external obliques and internal obliques.

See exercises
- *Four-point tummy vacuum (page 115)*
- *Supine lateral ball roll (page 125)*
- *Single arm cable pull (page 134)*

SCIATICA

Description

The sciatic nerve is the largest peripheral nerve in the body and runs from spinal nerves at L4 to S3 around the back of the hips and all the way down the legs. Sciatica is a painful condition caused by compression or irritation of one or more of the five spinal nerves that give rise to the sciatic nerve, or compression or irritation of the sciatic nerve itself. Those undertaking seated sports such as rowing and cycling are particularly vulnerable.

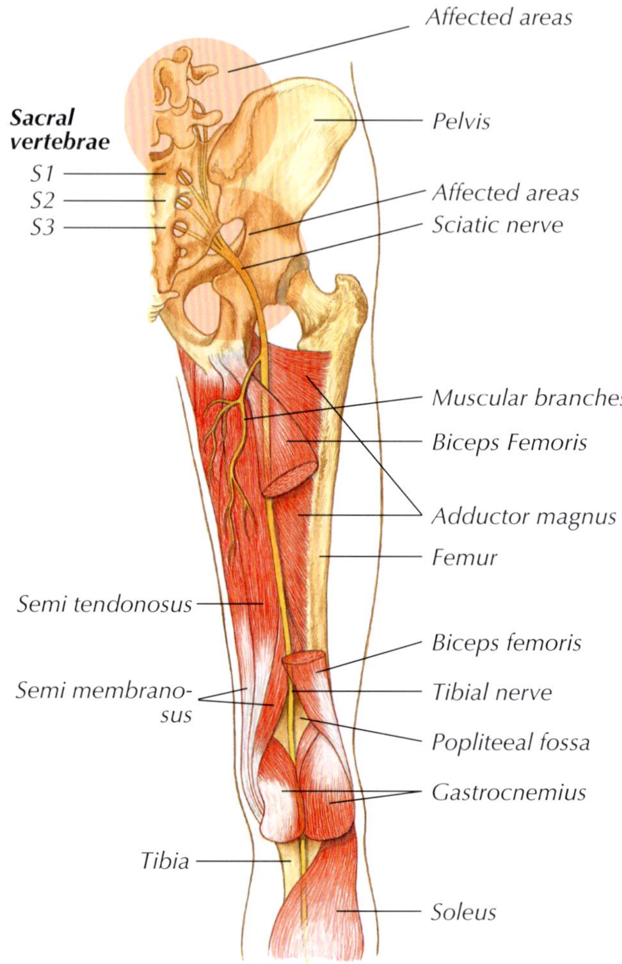

Symptoms

- Pain, tingling, aching pain or numbness.
- Pain may be felt in the lower back, gluteals, the hamstrings, calves and feet or a combination of these.

Causes

- Lumbar disc bulge.
- Spinal stenosis.
- Spondylolysthesis.
- Retrolysthesis.
- Piriformis syndrome.
- Core instability.
- Severe trauma to the lumbar spine.

Treatment

Acute

- Rest from normal sporting activities.
- Anti-inflammatory protocols.
- Neuromuscular Therapy™.
- Active Release Technique®.

Post-acute

- Heat treatments, contrast cold and hot.
- Corrective exercise, especially improving muscle balance in the lower limbs and lumbo-pelvic region, leading to gradual return to training (end-stage rehab) and competition.
- Surgery in extreme cases.

RECOVERY TIME WITH APPROPRIATE RECOVERY MANAGEMENT
3 to 6 weeks
Up to 3 months after surgery

Exercises

Stretching

- Any tight muscles around the pelvis, hip, knee or ankle joints and lumbar spine should be gradually and progressively stretched within pain-free ranges. These muscles will differ from person to person, but commonly include the hamstrings and lower abdominals.

Strengthening

- Strengthen any weak muscles around the lumbo-pelvic region. These muscles will differ from person to person, but commonly include the transversus abdominus, hip flexors, multifidus, psoas and lumbar erectors.

LUMBAR SPINE INJURIES

FACET JOINT PAIN

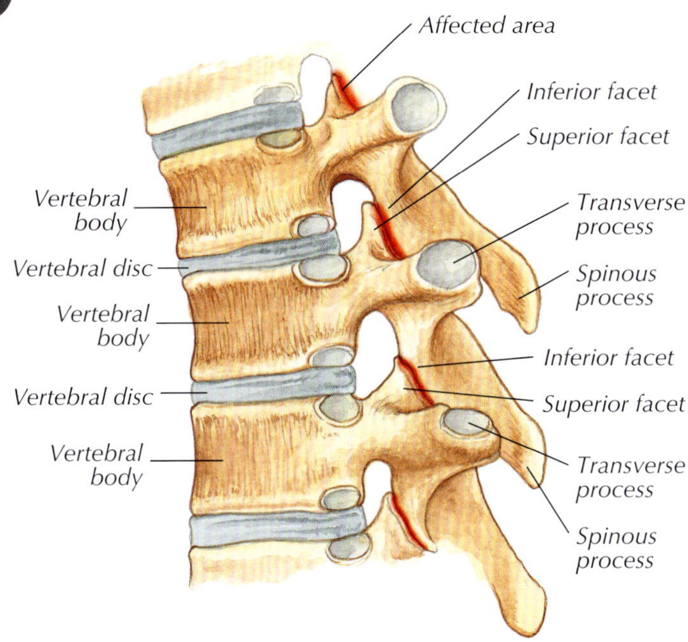

Description

The facet joints are synovial joints that help to limit movement of the spine and help vertebral bodies and discs to dissipate force. Facet joint pain may arise from the facet joint or from nerve compression. Sports that include repetitive lumbar extension such as cricket and gymnastics are particularly vulnerable.

Symptoms

- Persistent pain over the site of the inflamed joint.
- Muscle spasm around the affected area.
- Lumbar extension will normally exacerbate the symptoms.
- Pain occasionally radiates into the buttock and upper hamstring region.

Causes

- Hyper-lordotic lumbar spine – more than 35°, more common in females.
- Degenerative disc disease.
- Leg length discrepancy – functional (common) or structural (very rare).
- Core instability.
- Severe trauma to the lumbar spine.

Treatment

Acute

- Rest from normal sporting activities.
- Anti-inflammatory protocols.
- Sports massage.
- Neuromuscular Therapy™.

Post-acute

- Corrective exercise, especially improving muscle balance in the lower limbs and lumbo-pelvic region, leading to gradual return to training (end-stage rehab) and competition.

RECOVERY TIME WITH APPROPRIATE RECOVERY MANAGEMENT
3 to 6 weeks

Exercises

Stretching

- Any tight muscles around the pelvis, hip, knee or ankle joints should be gradually and progressively stretched within pain-free ranges. These muscles will differ from person to person, but commonly include the psoas, rectus femoris and lumbar erectors.

Strengthening

- Strengthen any weak muscles around the lumbo-pelvic region. These muscles will differ from person to person, but commonly include the transversus abdominus, gluteus maximus, hamstring groups and lower abdominals.

See exercises
- *Four-point tummy vacuum (page 115)*
- *Lower abdominals (page 123)*
- *Romanian deadlift (page 131)*

DISC DERANGEMENT NERVE ROOT COMPRESSION

Description

Between each vertebra in the spine lies a vertebral disc that has a nucleus pulposus in the middle and an annulus fibrosus around the outside. Due to pressure, particularly compression and torque, placed on the spine, the disc can bulge or herniate (where the nucleus perforates through the annulus), which may compress a spinal nerve root causing pain. However, it is possible to have a bulging disc without causing pain. The most common part of the disc to bulge or herniate is the posterior lateral part where it is not supported by the posterior longitudinal ligament. Seated sports such as rowing and cycling and sports that require spinal flexion and rotation, such as cricket, golf and baseball, are vulnerable.

Symptoms

- Mild to severe aching pain, tingling, muscular weakness, paralysis or numbness.
- Pain in lower back, gluteals, hamstrings, calves and feet or a combination of these.

Causes

- Poor lifting technique.
- High-speed repetitive lumbar flexion and rotation.
- Hypo-lordotic lumbar spine (less than 30°), caused by prolonged sitting.
- Hyper-lordotic lumbar spine (more than 35°) more common in females.
- Spinal stenosis.
- Spondylolysthesis.
- Retrolysthesis.
- Degenerative disc disease.

Disc herniation (central)

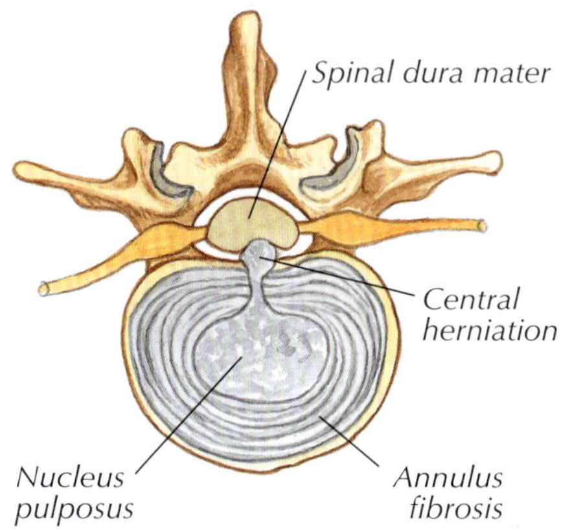

Disc bulge (lateral)

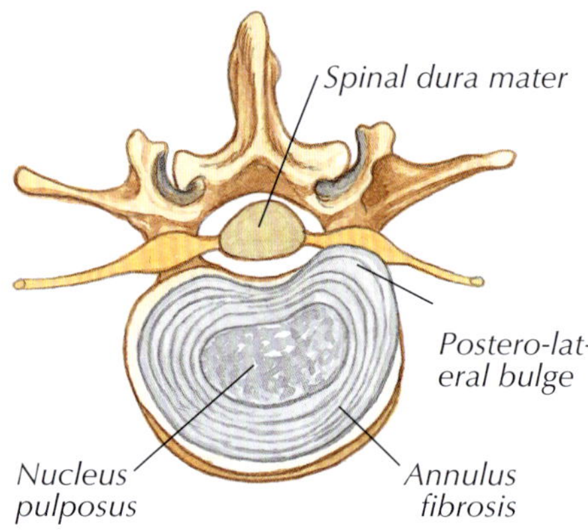

- Weak gluteus medius (lateral system).
- Leg length discrepancy – functional (common) or structural (very rare).
- Core instability.
- Severe trauma to the lumbar spine.

Treatment

Acute

- Rest from sporting activities.
- Anti-inflammatory protocols.
- Sports massage.
- Neuromuscular Therapy™.
- Active Release Technique®.

Post-acute

- Corrective exercise, especially improving muscle balance in lower limbs and lumbo-pelvic region, leading to gradual return to training (end-stage rehab) and competition.
- Surgery in extreme cases, such as a cauda equina.

Exercises

Stretching

- Any tight muscles around the pelvis, hip, knee or ankle joints should be gradually and progressively stretched within pain-free ranges. These muscles will differ from person to person, but commonly include the hamstrings and lower abdominals.

Strengthening

- Strengthen muscles around the lumbo-pelvic region. These will differ from person to person, but commonly include the transversus abdominus, multifidus, psoas and lumbar erectors.

RECOVERY TIME WITH APPROPRIATE RECOVERY MANAGEMENT
3 to 6 weeks

See exercises

- *McKenzie push-up (page 100)*
- *Four-point tummy vacuum (page 115)*
- *Hip and back extension (page 113)*

SPONDYLOLYSIS AND SPONDYLOLYSTHESIS

Description

Spondylolysis is a degenerative condition that leads to a fracture of the pars articularis, whereas spondylolysthesis is a complete break of the pars articularis and a forward slippage of the affected vertebra. Sports with repetitive lumbar extension such as cricket and gymnastics are vulnerable.

Symptoms

Spondylolysis

- Pain and/or muscle weakness around the affected area.
- Parasthesia in the lower back and/or the legs.
- Symptoms are often on one side.
- Stiffness and rigidity.
- Lumbar extension will normally exacerbate the symptoms.
- Pain occasionally radiates into the buttock and upper hamstring region.
- A hypo-lordotic lumbar spine and tight hamstrings may be a compensation caused by the injury.

Spondylolysthesis

- Forward slippage of the vertebra.
- Tightening of hamstring muscles.
- Abnormal gait.
- Gluteal atrophy (muscle wasting).
- Pain and/or muscle weakness around the affected area.
- Parasthesia and/or pain may radiate into the buttocks, hamstrings, calves and feet.
- Symptoms often just on one side.
- Stiffness and rigidity.
- Lumbar extension will normally exacerbate the symptoms.
- Sitting and attempting to stand may be painful.
- Coughing/sneezing can cause pain.

Spondylolysis

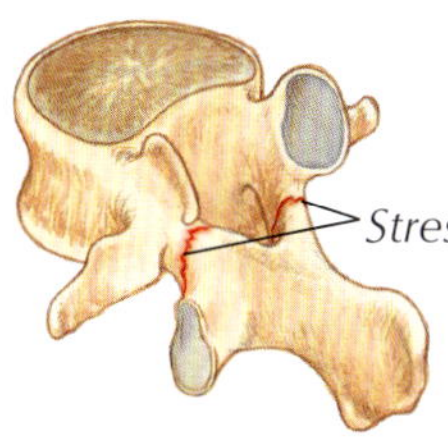

Causes

- Repetitive lumbar extension.
- Hyper-lordotic lumbar spine – more than 35°.
- Core instability.

Treatment

Acute

- Rest from sporting activities.
- Anti-inflammatory protocols.
- Sports massage.
- Neuromuscular Therapy™.

Post-acute

- Corrective exercise, especially improving muscle balance in the lower limbs and lumbo-pelvic region, leading to gradual return to training (end-stage rehab) and competition.
- Spondylolysthesis may require spinal fusion if conservative treatment is not effective.

RECOVERY TIME WITH APPROPRIATE RECOVERY MANAGEMENT
Can vary greatly from person to person; in some cases full recovery to sport may not be possible.

Spondylolysthesis
Side view of the lower spine and sacrum

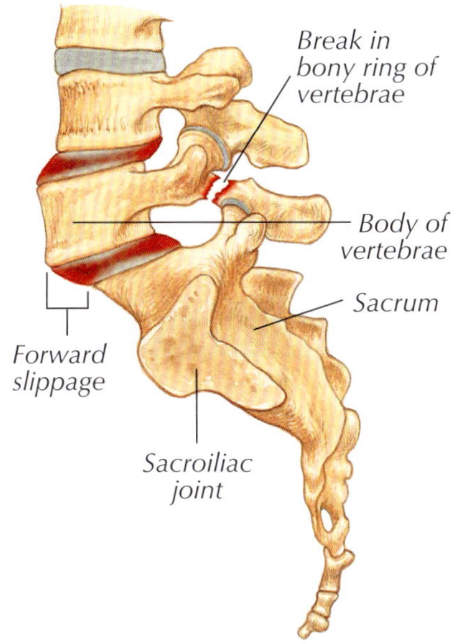

Exercises

Stretching

- Any tight muscles around the pelvis, hip, knee or ankle joints should be gradually and progressively stretched within pain-free ranges. Will differ from person to person. The hamstrings will often tighten to flatten the lumbar spine to avoid pain. Stretching the hamstrings could increase the likelihood of pain recurrence and should therefore be avoided or done with extreme caution.

Strengthening

- Strengthen any weak muscles around the lumbo-pelvic region. These muscles will differ from person to person. Exercises involving lumbar extension will exacerbate the symptoms and should be avoided.

See exercises
- *Four-point tummy vacuum (page 115)*
- *Lower abdominals (page 123)*
- *Supine hip extension on ball with belt (page 136)*

CERVICAL AND THORACIC SPINE INJURIES

ANKYLOSING SPONDYLITIS

Description

A chronic arthritic and auto-immune disease that causes the vertebrae to fuse together, ankylosing spondylitis normally causes stiffness in the region affected. It is more common in males than females and more prevalent amongst 20 to 40 year olds.

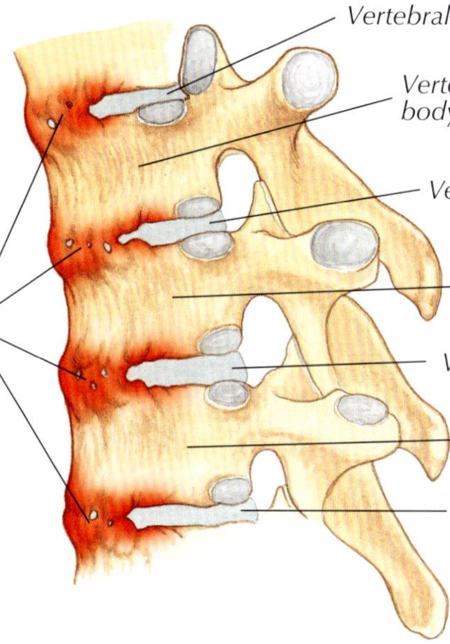

Symptoms

- Pain and stiffness in the spine and sacroiliac joints.
- Pain may radiate into the buttocks.
- Fatigue and nausea.
- Often associated with eye inflammation.
- Pre-pubescent sufferers may also suffer pain and swelling in the feet and ankles and may develop calcaneal bone spurs.

Causes

- Not fully understood, but believed to have a small genetic component.
- It is an auto-immune response.
- Some evidence exists to suggest an immune response to *Klebsiella* bacteria.

Treatment

- Sports massage.
- Improve/optimize muscle balance.
- Anti-inflammatory protocols.
- Anti-bacterial protocols.
- Low starch diet.

Exercises

Stretching

- Any tight muscles around neck, shoulders, upper back and upper torso. These muscles will differ from person to person.

Strengthening

- Strengthen any weak muscles around the neck, shoulders and upper back. These muscles will differ from person to person.

RECOVERY TIME WITH APPROPRIATE RECOVERY MANAGEMENT
Total recovery is currently not possible

See exercises
- *Four-point tummy vacuum (page 115)*
- *Lower abdominals (page 123)*
- *Single arm cable pull (page 134)*

ATLAS SUBLUXATION COMPLEX

Description

The Atlas Subluxation Complex (ASC) includes the measurable misalignment of the head, atlas and cervical spine, the contracted spinal musculature, postural distortion and short leg phenomena. The ASC includes the effects on the central and peripheral nervous system and the relationship to the symptoms and conditions directly related and those associated with this progressive degenerative condition. It occurs when the Atlas (C1 vertebra) is mis-aligned under the occipital region of the skull. Sports that involve trauma to the head and/or falls, such as soccer, downhill skiing, rugby, American football, boxing, martial arts, horse riding and motor racing are particularly vulnerable. ASC is more common than most realize and causes many so-called unrelated injuries.

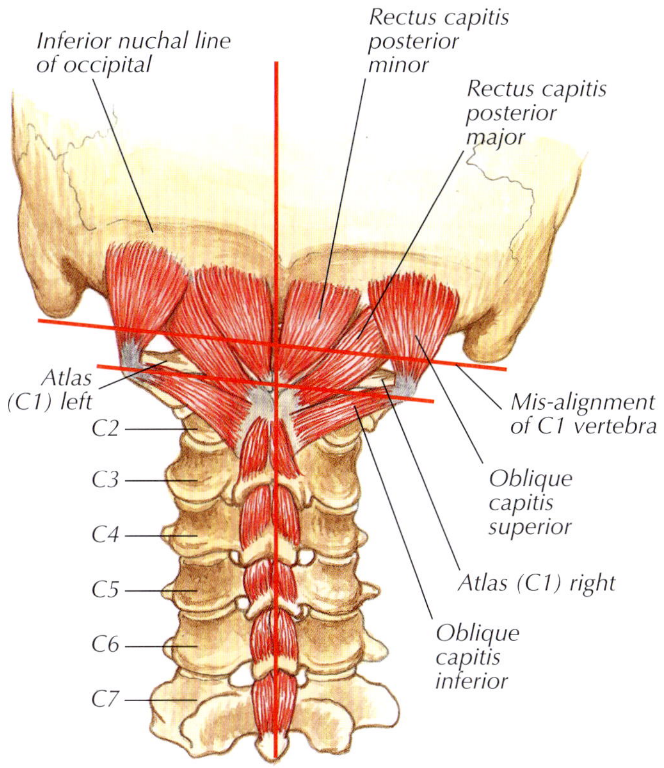

Symptoms

- May be asymptomatic (without symptoms).
- Functional leg-length discrepancy.
- Functional scoliosis.
- Possible pain in an assumedly unrelated injury.
- Possible pain and/or aching of the lower neck, upper back or lower back.
- Possible headaches.
- Possible Dowager's Hump.
- Possible sacroiliac joint dysfunction.
- Possible visceral irregularities.

RECOVERY TIME WITH APPROPRIATE RECOVERY MANAGEMENT
1 to 4 weeks

Causes

- Trauma to the head, neck or shoulder (including breaking a fall with the hand).
- Irregular breathing mechanics.
- Muscle imbalance in the jaw (temporomandibular joint).
- Eyesight irregularities.
- Vestibular irregularities.
- Unilateral structural foot and leg-length irregularity.

Treatment

- NUCCA chiropractic adjustment.
- Corrective exercise.
- May require correction of breathing, jaw mechanics, vision, vestibular, or structural leg-length discrepancy.

Exercises

Stretching

- Any tight muscles around neck, shoulders, upper back and upper torso. These muscles will differ from person to person.

Strengthening

- Strengthen any weak muscles around the neck, shoulders and upper back. These muscles will differ from person to person.

See exercises
- *Deep cervical flexors (page 119)*
- *Goof ball neck exercises (page 120)*
- *Single arm dumbbell shrug (page 133)*

SCHEUERMANN'S DISEASE

Description

This is a genetically related condition where the vertebrae of the spine grow (during childhood) with the anterior section smaller than the posterior section, creating a wedge shape. These wedge-shaped vertebrae cause a hyper-kyphotic posture of the spine ranging from minor to severe. Some people can perform their sport with little detriment while others can be unable to participate. It is more common in males than females.

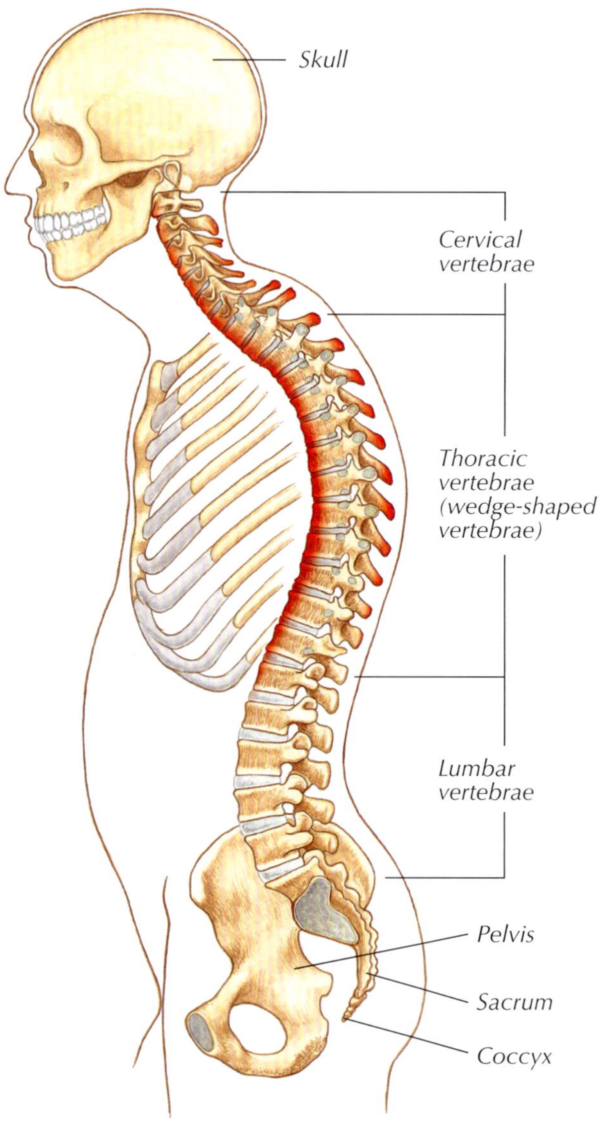

Symptoms

- Excessive curvature (hump) of the thoracic spine.
- Possible pain at the apex of the thoracic (spine) curve.
- 20–30% of sufferers also have scoliosis.
- Tight hamstrings are common.
- Possible, but rare organ damage.
- Possible, but rare nerve damage.

Causes

- Not fully understood, but widely believed to have a genetic component.

Treatment

- Sports massage.
- Joint manipulation (osteopath or chiropractor).
- Improve/optimize muscle balance.
- Stretching the abdominal and hamstring muscles.

RECOVERY TIME WITH APPROPRIATE RECOVERY MANAGEMENT

Total recovery is currently not possible

Exercises

Stretching

- Any tight muscles around neck, shoulders, upper back and upper torso. These muscles will differ from person to person.

Strengthening

- Strengthen any weak muscles around the neck, shoulders and upper back. These muscles will differ from person to person.

See exercises

- *Hamstrings – seated on Swiss ball (page 108)*
- *Four-point tummy vacuum (page 115)*
- *Lower abdominals (page 123)*

WHIPLASH

Description

Whiplash is an injury to the neck usually involving sudden distortion of the neck and often includes extension of the neck. It may result in neck muscle strain and/or a neck ligament sprain. It can also include damage to the nerves and/or fracture to the cervical vertebrae. Sports that involve collisions such as motor racing, horse riding, rugby, American football, skiing, ice hockey and soccer are particularly vulnerable.

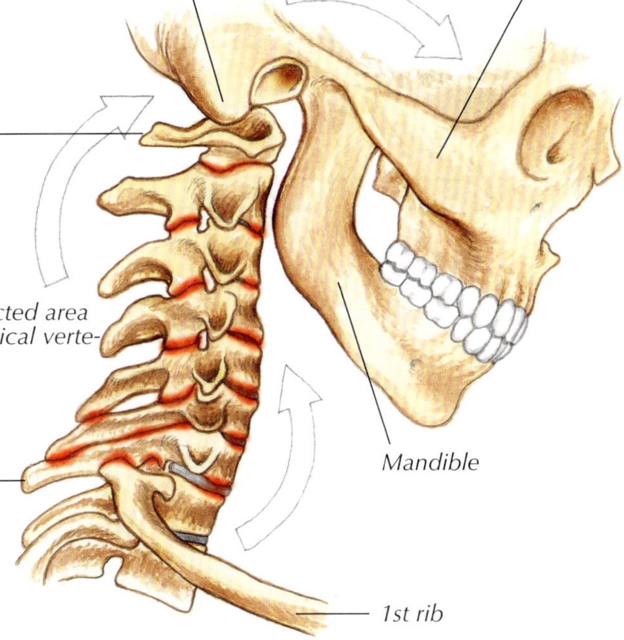

Symptoms

- Pain and/or aching of the neck and upper back, which may not appear immediately.
- Referred pain to the shoulders.
- Possible parasthesia in the arms.
- Headaches and/or dizziness.
- Possible blurred vision.
- Possible mandibular injury and dysfunction.

Causes

- Often due to a sudden flexion and extension of the cervical spine due to a collision, but can be a collision from any angle.

RECOVERY TIME WITH APPROPRIATE RECOVERY MANAGEMENT
3 days to 3 months

Treatment

Acute

- Seek medical treatment to check for fractures, nerve damage and concussion.
- Rest from normal sporting activities.
- Cold therapy in the first 24 hours.
- Anti-inflammatory protocols.

Post-acute

- Sports massage (after the acute phase).
- NUCCA chiropractic adjustment.
- Gradually increase range of motion of the neck in all ranges of movement in pain-free ranges.
- Corrective exercise, especially improving muscle balance in the upper body, leading to gradual return to training (end-stage rehab) and competition.

Exercises

Stretching

- Any tight muscles around neck, shoulders, upper back and upper torso and should be gradually and progressively stretched within pain-free ranges. These muscles will differ from person to person.

Strengthening

- Strengthen any weak muscles around the neck, shoulders and upper back. These muscles will differ from person to person.

See exercises
- *Deep cervical flexors (page 119)*
- *Goof ball neck exercises (page 120)*
- *Single arm dumbbell shrug (page 133)*

CHEST AND ABDOMINAL INJURIES

ABDOMINAL HERNIA

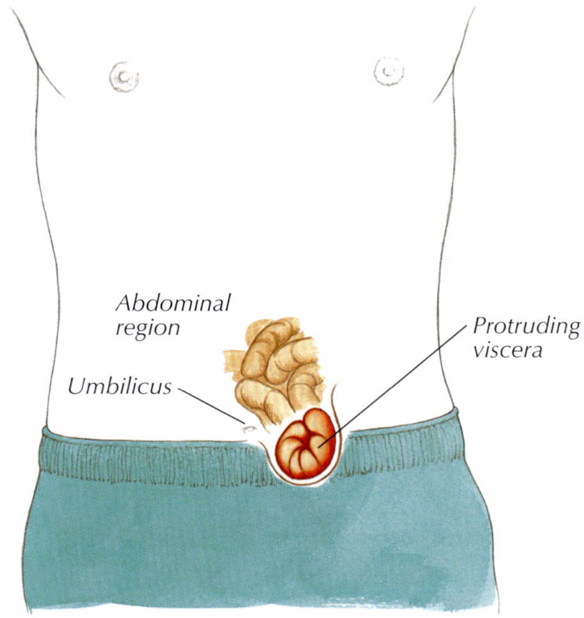

RECOVERY TIME WITH APPROPRIATE RECOVERY MANAGEMENT
6 to 8 weeks following surgery

Description

An abdominal hernia is a weakness in the abdominal wall that evolves into a localized hole through which adipose tissue or abdominal organs covered with peritoneum may protrude. An epigastric hernia usually appears in the region of the linea alba between the navel and the ribs. These occur mostly in men in their twenties. An umbilical hernia is a protrusion through the navel and usually occurs as a recurrence of the hernia from birth.

Symptoms

- Pain may or may not be present along the site of the hernia.
- A bulge in the abdominal region in the area of abdominal weakness.
- A protrusion of adipose tissue along the linea alba.
- A protrusion of intra-abdominal contents though the navel.

Causes

- Increased pressure in the compartment of the residing organ when the surrounding muscle is weakened.
- Pregnancy.
- Obesity.
- Scar tissue from previous surgery.
- Poor nutrition.
- Straining during bowel movements.
- Genetic factors.

Treatment

- Requires surgery followed by all stages of normal rehabilitation to end-stage rehab.

Exercises

Stretching

- Once the surgical wounds have healed, the torso should be gently moved into pain-free ranges of motion to recover the full range of motion of the spine and abdomen and to help re-align scar tissue.

Strengthening

- Once inflammation has ceased, strengthen the following muscles: transversus abdominus, internal obliques, external obliques and rectus abdominus.

See exercises
- *Four-point tummy vacuum (page 115)*
- *Lower abdominals (page 123)*
- *Wood chop (page 138)*

COSTOCHONDRITIS (TIETZE'S SYNDROME)

Description

Costal cartilage joins the first 10 ribs to the sternum. Costochondritis is a painful condition in the chest caused by inflammation of the costal cartilage. Adults between the ages of 20 and 40 seem to be more affected and rowers in particular seem to suffer this condition more than other athletes.

Symptoms

- Pain over the chest.
- Pain usually worsens due to exercise.
- Redness and swelling may be present
- Pain can be exacerbated by a deep inhalation.

Causes

- Repetitive micro-trauma to the chest.
- Trauma to the chest, such as the steering wheel hitting the chest in a car accident.
- Upper respiratory infections have also been implicated with this condition.

Treatment

Acute

- Rest from normal activities that exacerbate the symptoms.
- Anti-inflammatory protocols.

Post-acute

- Heat therapy.

RECOVERY TIME WITH APPROPRIATE RECOVERY MANAGEMENT

- 4 weeks to 6 months

Exercises

Stretching

- No specific stretches will aid healing.

Strengthening

- No specific exercises will aid healing.

Sites of injury shown in red

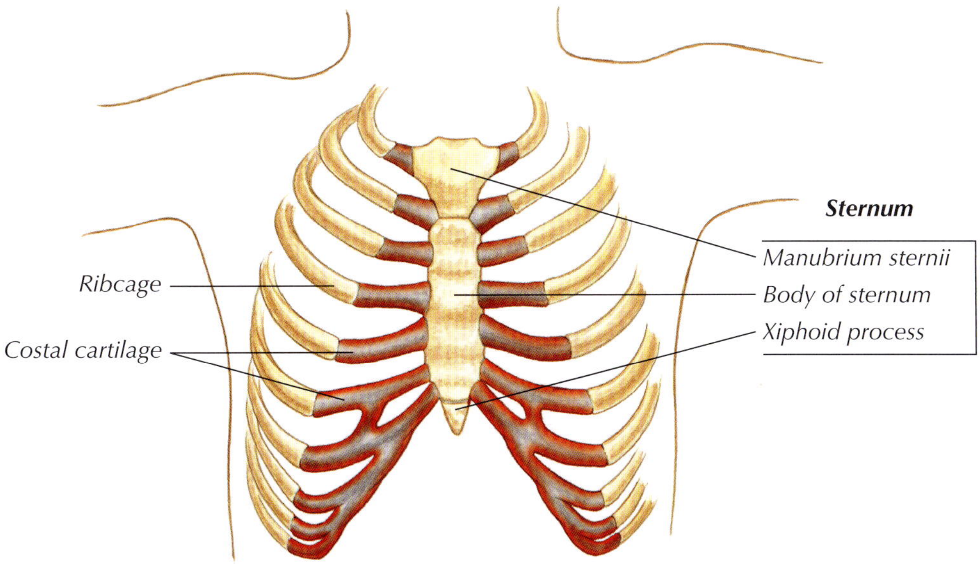

PECTORALIS MAJOR STRAIN

Description

The pectoralis major muscle originates on the sternum, medial half of the clavicle and the costal cartilage of the first six ribs and inserts onto the greater tubercle of the humerus. This injury is either a grade 1, 2 or 3 tear of the pectoralis major muscle and occurs almost exclusively in males between the ages of 20 and 50.

Symptoms

- Pain in the chest and upper arm.
- Weakness in the affected arm.
- Bruising.
- Dimpling when there is a total rupture.

Causes:

- Forceful activities such as weight-lifting, especially bench pressing.
- Blocking and tackling in contact sports
- Steroid use has been shown to increase the risk.

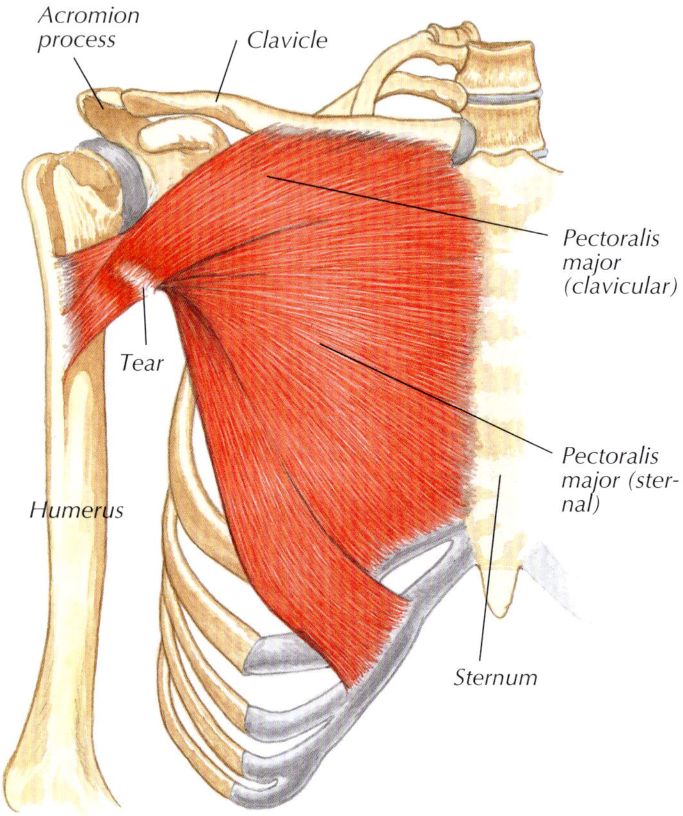

Treatment

Acute

- Use RICE (see page 29) in the first 24 to 48 hours to prevent further damage and optimize healing time.
- Anti-inflammatory protocols.

Post-acute

- Sports massage.
- Corrective exercise, especially improving muscle balance in the upper body, leading to gradual return to training (end-stage rehab) and competition to prevent re-injury.
- Strength training normally begins with isometric, then concentric and finally eccentric work is added.
- Surgery may be required for grade 3 tears.

RECOVERY TIME WITH APPROPRIATE RECOVERY MANAGEMENT
Grade 1: Days
Grade 2: 3 to 6 weeks
Grade 3: 2 to 3 months

Exercises

Stretching

- A gradual and pain-free increase in range of motion of the shoulder joint.
- Any tight muscles around neck, shoulders, upper back and upper torso. These muscles will differ from person to person.

Strengthening

- Strengthen any weak muscles around the neck, shoulders and upper back. These muscles will differ from person to person.

See exercises
- *Horse stance vertical (page 122)*
- *Single arm cable push (page 132)*

RIB FRACTURE

Description
A fracture to one of the 12 ribs, this is a relatively common injury in contact sports caused by a blow to the ribs from a fist or elbow or by landing forcibly on a hard surface such as the ground. Players of rugby, American football, boxing and martial arts are particularly vulnerable to this injury.

Symptoms
- Pain and swelling over the site of the fracture.
- Difficulty breathing.
- Pain with coughing and sneezing.

Causes
- Trauma to the rib cage.
- A punch, elbow or kick to the ribs.
- A fall on hard ground landing on the rib cage.

Treatment
- Rest is all that can be done.
- Requires medical attention.

RECOVERY TIME WITH APPROPRIATE RECOVERY MANAGEMENT
3 to 12 weeks

Exercises
Stretching
- None applicable.

Strengthening
- No specific exercises will aid the healing.
- Strengthening of the core muscles may help prevent future injury to the ribs, once the injury has healed.

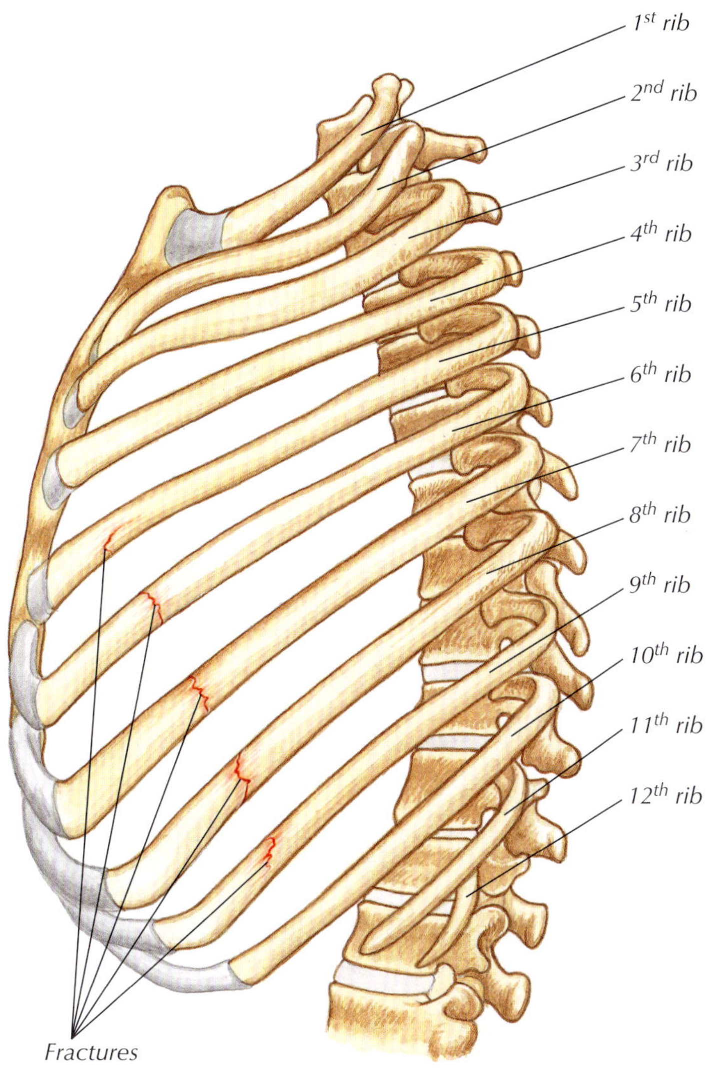

See exercises
- *Four-point tummy vacuum (page 115)*
- *Wood chop (page 138)*
- *Deadlift (page 127)*

STERNOCLAVICULAR JOINT SPRAIN

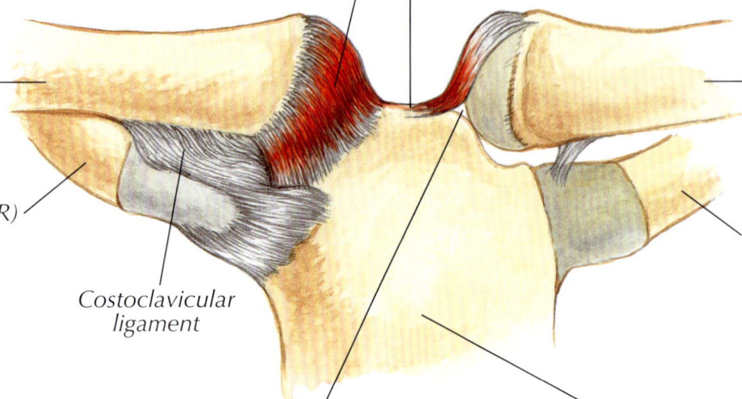

Description

The sternoclavicular (SC) joint is a synovial joint connecting the sternum and clavicle; it is divided by an articular disc and held together by four ligaments. An SC joint sprain is a grade 1, 2 or 3 sprain of one or more of the ligaments surrounding the joint. Sports that involve trauma to the torso and/or falls, such as soccer, downhill skiing, rugby, American football, boxing, martial arts, horse riding and motor racing are more vulnerable.

Symptoms

- Pain with palpation over the site of the joint.
- Pain radiating into the shoulder joint.

Causes

- Trauma to the torso or shoulder.
- Breaking a fall with the hand.

Treatment

- Rest from normal training.
- Seek medical advice as the joint is very close to important blood vessels.

RECOVERY TIME WITH APPROPRIATE RECOVERY MANAGEMENT
3 to 4 weeks

Exercises

Stretching

- When able, the shoulder should be moved gently into pain-free ranges of motion to recover the full range of motion of the spine and abdomen and to help re-align scar tissue.

Strengthening

- No specific exercises will aid the healing.
- Closed-chain shoulder exercises are a good place to start the rehabilitation process.

See exercises
- *Horse stance vertical (page 122)*

SHOULDER INJURIES

ACROMIOCLAVICULAR JOINT SPRAIN

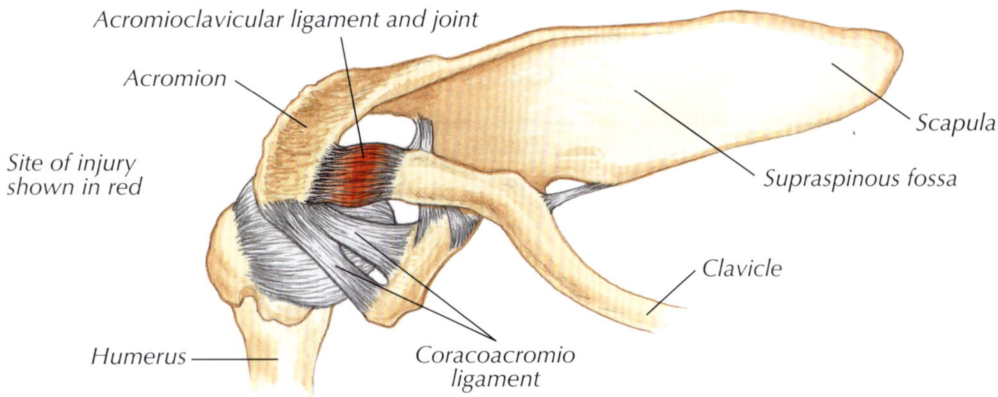

Description

The acromioclavicular (AC) joint is a gliding synovial joint connecting the acromion of the scapula to the clavicle, and is held together by three ligaments. An AC joint sprain is a grade 1, 2 or 3 sprain of one or more of the ligaments surrounding the joint. Sports that involve trauma to the torso and/or falls, such as soccer, downhill skiing, rugby, American football, boxing, martial arts, horse riding and motor racing are more vulnerable.

Symptoms

- Pain with palpation over the site of the joint.
- Pain around the whole shoulder joint.
- Possible swelling.

Causes

- Trauma to the torso or shoulder.
- Breaking a fall with the hand.

Treatment

- Rest from normal training.
- Initially the arm may need to be immobilized in a sling.
- Taping.
- Anti-inflammatory protocols.
- Surgery may be required for a total rupture.

RECOVERY TIME WITH APPROPRIATE RECOVERY MANAGEMENT
3 weeks to 4 months

Exercises

Stretching

- When able, the shoulder should be moved gently into pain-free ranges of motion to recover the full range of motion of the spine and abdomen and help re-align scar tissue.

Strengthening

- No specific exercises will aid the healing.
- Closed-chain shoulder exercises are a good place to start the rehabilitation process.

See exercises
- *Pectoralis minor (page 110)*
- *Prone cobra (page 114)*
- *Horse stance vertical (page 122)*

BICEPS BRACHII STRAIN

Description

The biceps brachii muscle originates from the coracoid process and supra glenoid tubercle of the scapula and inserts into the tuberosity of the radius and aponeurosis of the biceps brachii. Biceps brachii strain is a grade 1, 2 or 3 tear to one of those muscles or tendons. The most common injury is to the proximal tendon of the long head. Rotator cuff strains and labrum tears may occur at the same time. Athletes who regularly perform heavy weightlifting as part of their training or competition are particularly vulnerable.

Symptoms

- Sudden, sharp pain in the upper arm.
- A snap may be heard.
- Pain on palpation of the affected area.
- Weakness of the affected limb.
- Bunching of the muscle may be observed with a complete rupture.

Causes

- Heavy weightlifting – putting excessive loading through the elbow joint.
- Upper cross syndrome (see glossary page 141).
- Impingement of the biceps tendon against the acromion.

Treatment

Acute

- RICE (see page 29).
- Anti-inflammatory protocols.

Post-acute

- Sports massage.
- Gradual increase of range of motion of the shoulder and elbow within pain-free ranges.
- Corrective exercise, especially improving muscle balance in the upper body, leading to gradual return to training (end-stage rehab) and competition to prevent re-injury.
- Strength training normally begins with isometric, then concentric and finally eccentric work is added.
- Surgery may be required with a total rupture.

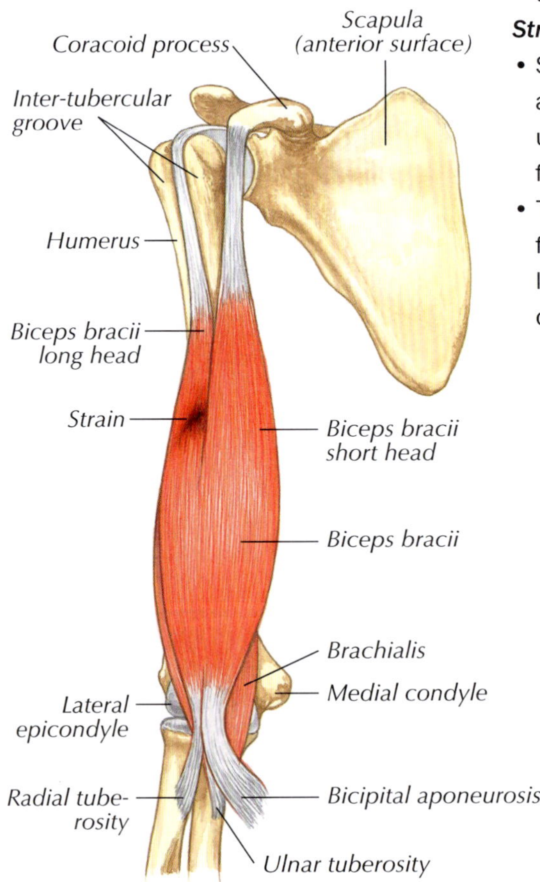

RECOVERY TIME WITH APPROPRIATE RECOVERY MANAGEMENT
Grade 1: Days
Grade 2: 3 to 6 weeks
Grade 3: 2 to 3 months

Exercises

Stretching

- A gradual and pain-free increase in range of motion of the shoulder joint.
- Any tight muscles around neck, shoulders, upper back and upper torso. These muscles will differ from person to person, however, the pectoralis minor is commonly tight.

Strengthening

- Strengthen any weak muscles around the neck, shoulders and upper back. These muscles will differ from person to person.
- The rhomboids, trapezius (middle fibers), teres minor, infraspinatus, longus colli and longus capitis are often weak.

See exercises
- *Prone cobra (page 114)*
- *Horse stance vertical (page 122)*
- *Cable rotator cuff training (page 116)*

DISLOCATION

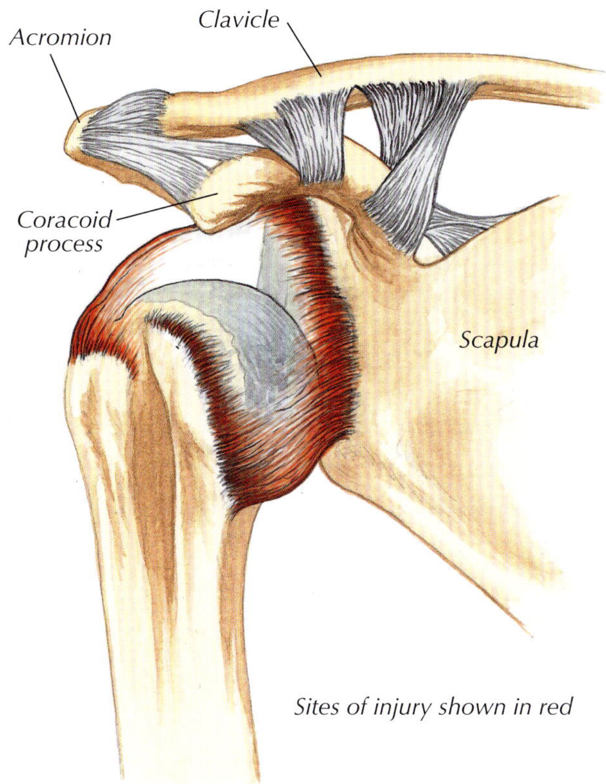

Description

A shoulder dislocation occurs when the head of the humerus separates from the scapula at the glenohumeral joint. A dislocation can be anterior (95%), posterior (4%) or inferior (1%). The shoulder joint is the most mobile and least stable joint in the body and is the most commonly dislocated. The joint capsule, ligaments, bone, blood vessels, nerves and tendons are often damaged at the same time as the dislocation. Sports that involve trauma to the torso such as soccer, downhill skiing, rugby, American football, boxing, martial arts, horse riding and motor racing are more vulnerable to this injury.

Symptoms

- Significant pain around the shoulder.
- Immobilization of the affected arm.
- Visibly displaced shoulder.
- Possible numbness of the affected arm.

Causes

- Trauma to the torso or shoulder.
- Breaking a fall with the hand, especially with abduction and external rotation of the shoulder.

Treatment

Acute

- Surgery is normally required.
- Rest from normal training.
- Initially the arm may need to be immobilized in a sling.
- Taping.
- Anti-inflammatory protocols.

Post-acute

- Gradual increase in range of motion of the shoulder within pain-free ranges.
- Corrective exercise, especially improving muscle balance in the upper body, leading to gradual return to training (end-stage rehab) and competition to prevent re-injury.
- Strength training normally begins with isometric, then concentric and finally eccentric work is added.

RECOVERY TIME WITH APPROPRIATE RECOVERY MANAGEMENT
3 to 4 months

Exercises

Stretching

- When able, the shoulder should be moved gently into pain-free ranges of motion to recover the full range of motion of the spine and abdomen and help re-align scar tissue.

Strengthening

- No specific exercises will aid the healing.
- Closed-chain shoulder exercises are a good place to start the rehabilitation process, progressing on to open chain.

See exercises
- *Shoulder mobilization in all planes (page 103)*
- *Horse stance vertical (page 122)*
- *Cable rotator cuff training (page 116)*

FRACTURE OF THE CLAVICLE

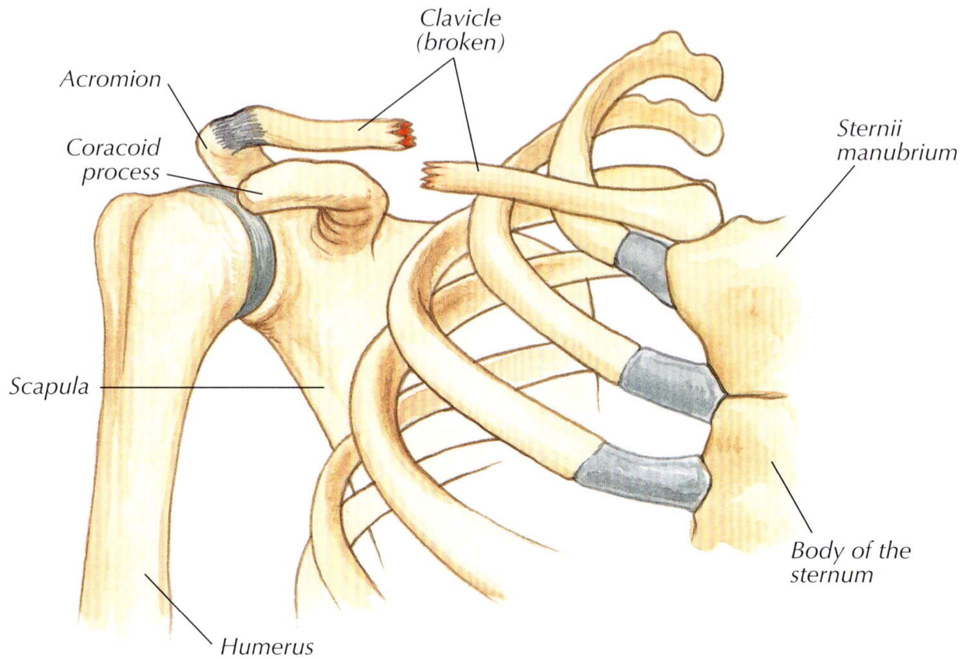

Description

This injury is a fracture to one of the clavicles (collar bones), caused by a blow to the clavicle, by landing forcibly on the shoulder or by breaking a fall with an outstretched arm. Sports such as rugby, ice hockey and American football are particularly vulnerable.

Symptoms

- Severe pain.
- Swelling over the site of the fracture.
- Possible deformity may be seen.

Causes

- Trauma to the clavicle.
- A fall on hard ground landing on the shoulder.
- Breaking a fall with an outstretched arm.

Treatment

- Rest.
- Immobilization of the affected limb in a sling for one to two weeks.
- Anti-inflammatory protocols and pain relief.
- Surgery may be required in some instances.

RECOVERY TIME WITH APPROPRIATE RECOVERY MANAGEMENT
3 to 4 weeks

Exercises

Stretching

- After one to two weeks, a gradual and pain-free increase in range of motion of the shoulder joint in all planes of motion.
- Any tight muscles around neck, shoulders, upper back and upper torso. These muscles will differ from person to person, however, the pectoralis minor is commonly tight.

Strengthening

- Strengthen any weak muscles around the neck, shoulders and upper back. These muscles will differ from person to person.

See exercises
- *Shoulder mobilization in all planes (page 103)*
- *Horse stance vertical (page 122)*

FROZEN SHOULDER

Description

Frozen shoulder is a painful condition due to inflammation of the shoulder capsule, which stiffens and prevents normal movement of the shoulder joint. It is more common in people over 40 years old and in females. Risk factors also include diabetes, stroke, lung disease and heart disease.

RECOVERY TIME WITH APPROPRIATE RECOVERY MANAGEMENT
3 to 12 months

Symptoms

- Aching pain and weakness in the affected shoulder.
- Range of motion in the shoulder will be severely limited.
- Inability to carry out normal activities.
- Pain when lying on the affected side, affecting sleep.
- Muscular atrophy.

Causes

- A previous injury to the shoulder.
- Recent surgery to the shoulder.
- Rheumatic disease.

Treatment

Acute

- Anti-inflammatory protocols.
- Sports massage.
- Acupuncture.

Post-acute

- Heat therapy.
- Gradual increase in range of motion of the shoulder within pain-free ranges.
- May require manipulation under anesthetic.
- Corrective exercise, especially improving muscle balance in the upper body, leading to gradual return to training (end-stage rehab) and competition to prevent re-injury.
- Strength training normally begins with isometric, then concentric and finally eccentric work is added.
- Surgery may be required in extreme cases.

Exercises

Stretching

- A gradual and pain-free increase in range of motion of the shoulder joint.
- Any tight muscles around neck, shoulders, upper back and upper torso.

Strengthening

- Strengthen any weak muscles around the neck, shoulders and upper back. These muscles will differ from person to person.

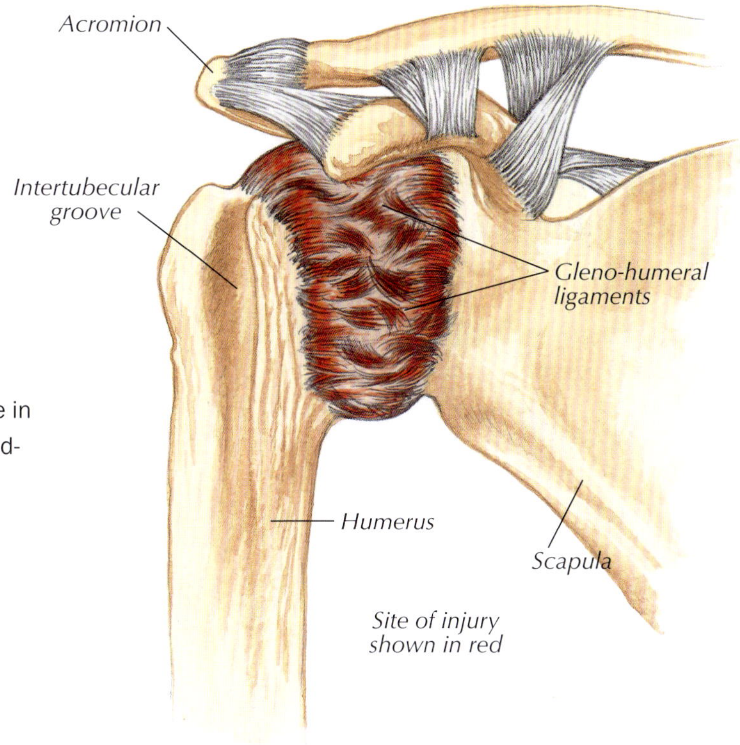

See exercises
• *Shoulder mobilization in all planes (page 103)*

GLENOID LABRUM TEAR

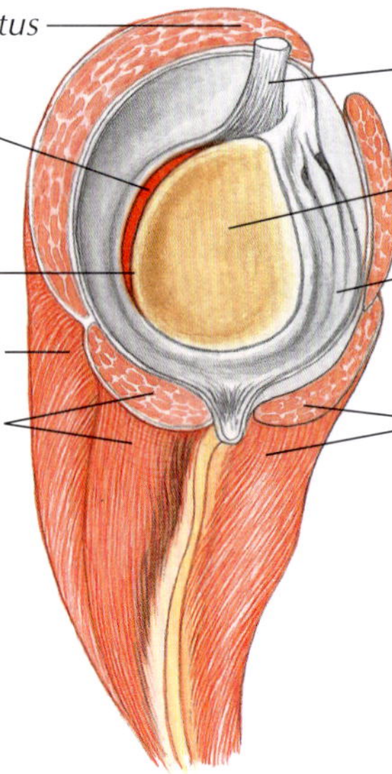

Description

The glenoid labrum is a fibro cartilaginous rim attached around the glenoid cavity of the scapula. A labral tear can occur in ten different ways, and overhead sports such as baseball, racket sports, cricket, volleyball and swimming are most vulnerable.

Symptoms

- A dull, throbbing ache around the shoulder.
- Difficulty sleeping due to shoulder pain.
- Weakness of the affected limb.
- A sensation of 'catching or 'pinching' may be felt.
- Over-arm activities will often exacerbate the symptoms.
- Range of motion of the shoulder may be limited.

Causes

- Repetitive, high velocity over-arm sports.
- Upper cross syndrome.
- Shoulder joint instability.
- Trauma to the shoulder, including dislocation.
- Biceps brachii injury.

Treatment

Acute

- Surgery may be required to repair the labrum.
- Rest from overhead activities.
- Anti-inflammatory protocols.

Post-acute

- Sports massage.
- Taping.
- Gradual increase in range of motion of the shoulder within pain-free ranges.
- Corrective exercise, especially improving muscle balance in the upper body, leading to gradual return to training (end-stage rehab) and competition to prevent re-injury.
- Strength training normally begins with isometric, then concentric and finally eccentric work is added.

RECOVERY TIME WITH APPROPRIATE RECOVERY MANAGEMENT
Up to one year following surgery

Exercises

Stretching

- A gradual and pain-free increase in range of motion of the shoulder joint.
- Any tight muscles around neck, shoulders, upper back and upper torso. These muscles will differ from person to person, however, the pectoralis minor is commonly tight.

Strengthening

- Strengthen any weak muscles around the neck, shoulders and upper back. These muscles will differ from person to person.
- Gradual loading of the joint, beginning with closed-chain exercises.
- The rhomboids, trapezius (middle fibres), teres minor, infraspinatus, longus colli and longus capitis are often weak.

See exercises
- *Prone cobra (page 114)*
- *Horse stance vertical (page 122)*
- *Cable rotator cuff training (page 116)*

IMPINGEMENT SYNDROME (SWIMMER/THROWER'S SHOULDER)

Description

Impingement syndrome occurs when the rotator cuff tendons become impinged between the acromion process of the scapula and the head of the humerus. Continued impingement leads to inflammation and tenderness of the rotator cuff tendons. If impingement syndrome continues, it can lead to rotator cuff strain. Overhead sports such as baseball, racket sports, cricket, volleyball and swimming are more vulnerable.

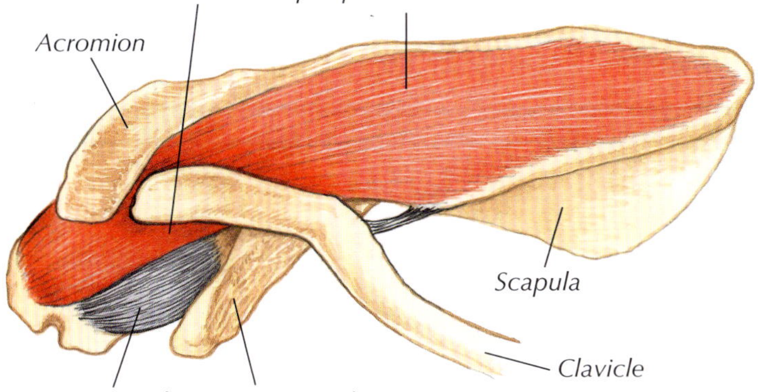

Symptoms

- Pain, weakness and loss of movement in the affected arm.
- Over-arm activities will exacerbate the symptoms.
- Range of motion in the shoulder may be limited.

Causes

- Upper cross syndrome.
- Bone spurs.
- Shoulder joint instability.

RECOVERY TIME WITH APPROPRIATE RECOVERY MANAGEMENT
3 to 6 weeks

Treatment

Acute

- Rest from overhead activities.
- Anti-inflammatory protocols.

Post-acute

- Sports massage.
- Taping.
- Gradual increase in range of motion of the shoulder within pain-free ranges.
- Corrective exercise, especially improving muscle balance in the upper body, leading to gradual return to training (end-stage rehab) and competition to prevent re-injury.
- Strength training normally begins with isometric, then concentric and finally eccentric work is added.
- Surgery may be required to remove bone spurs.

Exercises

Stretching

- A gradual and pain-free increase in range of motion of the shoulder joint.
- Any tight muscles around neck, shoulders, upper back and upper torso. These muscles will differ from person to person, however, the pectoralis minor is commonly tight.

Strengthening

- Strengthen any weak muscles around the neck, shoulders and upper back. These muscles will differ from person to person.
- The rhomboids, trapezius (middle fibers), teres minor, infraspinatus, longus colli and longus capitis are often weak.

See exercises
- *Pectoralis minor stretch (page 110)*
- *Prone cobra (page 114)*
- *Horse stance vertical (page 122)*

ROTATOR CUFF STRAIN

Description

The rotator cuff muscles include the supraspinatus, subscapularis, teres minor and infraspinatus. A strain can be a grade 1, 2 or 3 tear to one of the rotator cuff muscles or tendons, although it is more common to injure the tendons with the supraspinatus the most commonly injured muscle. Rotator cuff strains are a common shoulder injury, with overhead sports such as baseball, racket sports, cricket, volleyball and swimming the more vulnerable sports.

Symptoms

- Pain around the region of the lateral shoulder.
- Pain when raising the arm.
- Weakness of the affected limb.
- Over-arm activities will often exacerbate the symptoms.
- Range of motion of the shoulder may be limited.

Causes

- Upper cross syndrome.
- Bone spurs.
- Shoulder joint instability.

Treatment

Acute

- Rest from overhead activities.
- Anti-inflammatory protocols.

Post-acute

- Sports massage.
- Taping.
- Gradual increase in range of motion in the shoulder within pain-free ranges.
- Corrective exercise, especially improving muscle balance in the upper body, leading to gradual return to training (end-stage rehab) and competition to prevent re-injury.
- Strength training normally begins with isometric, then concentric and finally eccentric work is added.
- Surgery may be required to remove bone spurs.

Exercises

Stretching

- A gradual and pain-free increase in range of motion in shoulder joint.
- Any tight muscles around neck, shoulders, upper back and upper torso. These muscles will differ from person to person, however, the pectoralis minor is commonly tight.

Strengthening

- Strengthen any weak muscles around the neck, shoulders and upper back. These muscles will differ from person to person.
- The rhomboids, trapezius (middle fibers), teres minor, infraspinatus, longus colli and longus capitis are often weak.

RECOVERY TIME WITH APPROPRIATE RECOVERY MANAGEMENT
Grade 1: Days
Grade 2: 3 to 6 weeks
Grade 3: 2 to 3 months

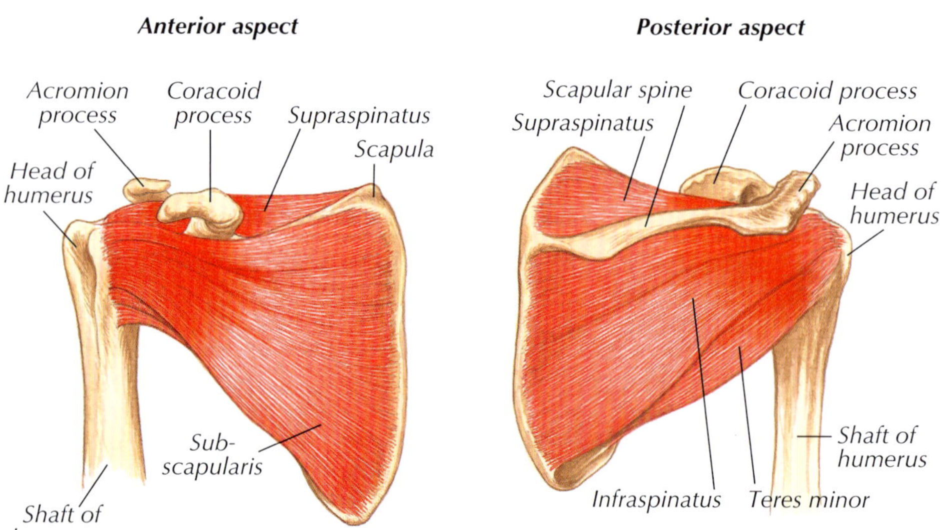

Sites of injury shown in darker red

See exercises
- *Prone cobra (page 114)*
- *Horse stance vertical (page 122)*
- *Cable rotator cuff training (page 116)*

ELBOW INJURIES

MEDIAL EPICONDYLITIS (GOLFER'S ELBOW)

Description

This is a painful condition of the wrist flexor tendons as they attach to the medial epicondyle of the humerus. It is believed that repetitive over-use of the arm causes micro-trauma to the common flexor tendon over time. While the condition does affect golfers, it can affect almost any sport, especially throwing sports such as baseball and cricket.

Symptoms

- Pain around the medial epicondyle region.
- Pain radiating down the forearm when gripping objects.

Causes

- Repetitive overuse of the arm.
- Rapid deceleration of the elbow during throwing sports.
- Direct trauma to the medial epicondyle of the humerus.
- Rapid increase in volume of sport.

Treatment

Acute

- Rest from normal activities/training.
- Ice in the first 24 to 48 hours.
- Anti-inflammatory protocols.

Post-acute

- Heat therapy.
- Sports massage.
- Active Release Technique®.
- Gradual increase in range of motion in the wrist and elbow within pain-free ranges.
- Corrective exercise, especially improving muscle balance in the upper body, leading to gradual return to training (end-stage rehab) and competition to prevent re-injury.
- Strength training normally begins with isometric, then concentric and finally eccentric work is added.

RECOVERY TIME WITH APPROPRIATE RECOVERY MANAGEMENT
3 weeks to 3 months

Exercises

Stretching

- A gradual and pain-free increase in range of motion of the wrist and elbow joints.
- Any tight muscles around neck, shoulders, upper back and upper torso. These muscles will differ from person to person.

Strengthening

- Strengthen any weak muscles around the neck, shoulders and upper back. These muscles will differ from person to person.
- The forearm flexors should be strengthened isometrically, concentrically and eccentrically.

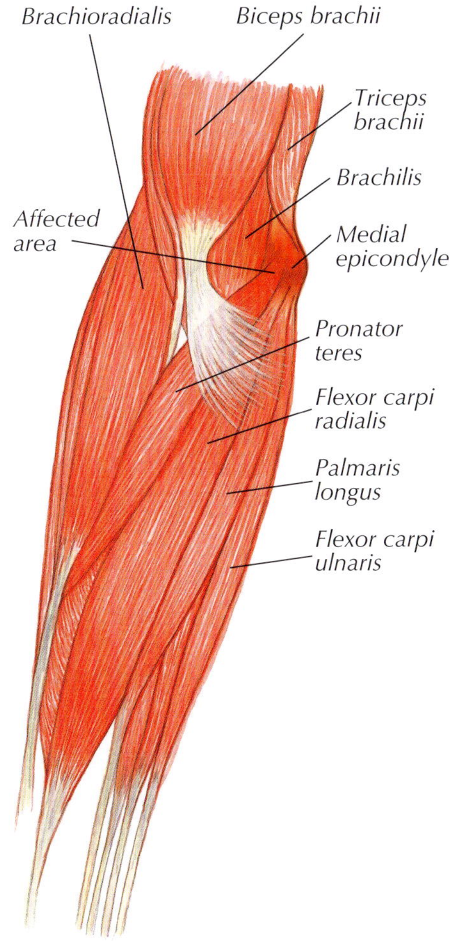

See exercises
- *Wrist flexors (page 140)*
- *Medicine ball shoulder internal rotators (page 130)*

MEDIAN NERVE ENTRAPMENT

Description

Entrapment or compression of the median nerve as it passes the elbow joint by the ligament of Struthers (very rare), the bicipital aponeurosis or by the two heads of the pronator teres muscle. If not treated early enough, this can lead to permanent paralysis of the arm and hand.

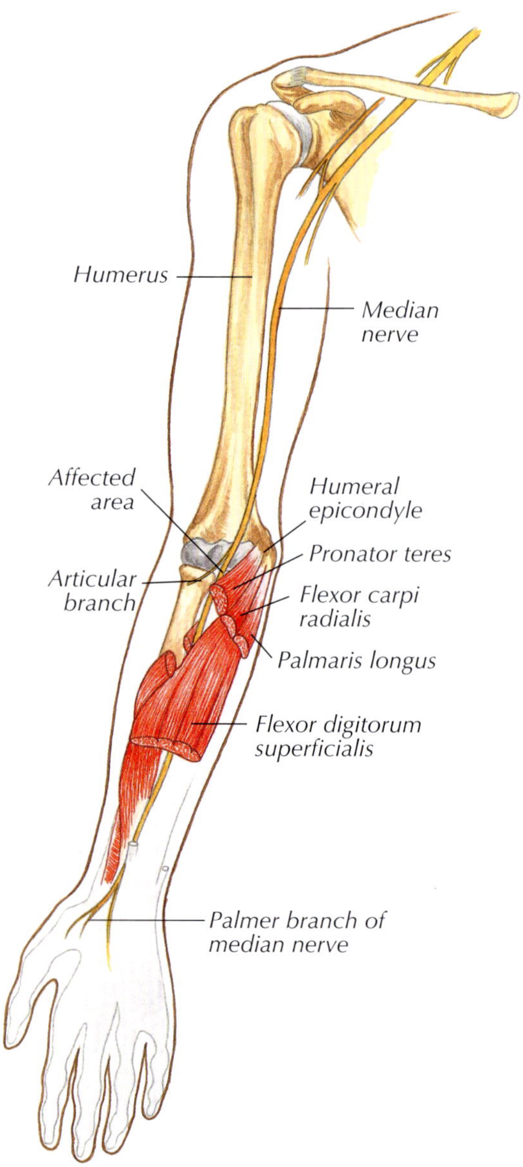

Symptoms

- Tenderness and a dull, achy pain in the wrist flexor muscle region.
- Pain, numbness and tingling along the forearm and possibly into the wrist and hand.
- Possible atrophy of the thenar eminence.

Causes

- Muscular, tendon or ligamentous inflammation.
- Abnormal bone growths, tumours and other space-occupying lesions.

Treatment

Acute

- Rest from activities that exacerbate the condition.
- Ice therapy.
- Anti-inflammatory protocols.
- Sports massage.
- Active Release Technique®.

Post-acute

- Gradual increase in range of motion in the wrist and elbow within pain-free ranges.
- Corrective exercise, especially improving muscle balance in the upper body, leading to gradual return to training (end-stage rehab) and competition to prevent re-injury.
- Strength training normally begins with isometric, then concentric and finally eccentric work is added. The forearm muscles may need strengthening.
- May require surgery in extreme cases.

RECOVERY TIME WITH APPROPRIATE RECOVERY MANAGEMENT
6 to 12 weeks

Exercises

Stretching

- A gradual and pain-free increase in range of motion of the wrist and elbow joints.
- The median nerve will require mobilizing (flossing).
- Stretch any tight muscles around neck, shoulders, upper back and upper torso. These muscles will differ from person to person.

Strengthening

- Strengthen any weak muscles around the neck, shoulders and upper back. These muscles will differ from person to person.
- The forearm flexors, supinators and pronators should be strengthened isometrically, concentrically and eccentrically.

See exercises

- *Median nerve mobilization (page 101)*
- *Wrist flexors (page 140)*
- *Single-arm cable push (page 132)*

RADIAL NERVE ENTRAPMENT (RADIAL TUNNEL SYNDROME)

Description

This condition can be confused with tennis elbow. Caused by entrapment or compression of the radial nerve as it passes the lateral epicondyle by inflamed muscles and tendons. Direct trauma to the lateral epicondyle may damage the radial nerve.

Symptoms

- Tenderness and a dull, achy pain in the wrist extensor muscle region.
- Tingling and numbness.
- Pain worsens with supination under load.

Causes

- Inflammation of the muscles surrounding the radial tunnel.
- Direct blow to the outside of the elbow.

Treatment

Acute

- Rest from activities that exacerbate the condition, especially wrist extension, supination and pronation.
- Ice therapy.
- Anti-inflammatory protocols.
- Sports massage.
- Active Release Technique®.

Post-acute

- Gradual increase of range of motion of the wrist and elbow within pain-free ranges.
- Corrective exercise, especially improving muscle balance in the upper body, leading to gradual return to training (end-stage rehab) and competition to prevent re-injury.
- Strength training normally begins with isometric, then concentric and finally eccentric work is added. The forearm muscles may need strengthening.

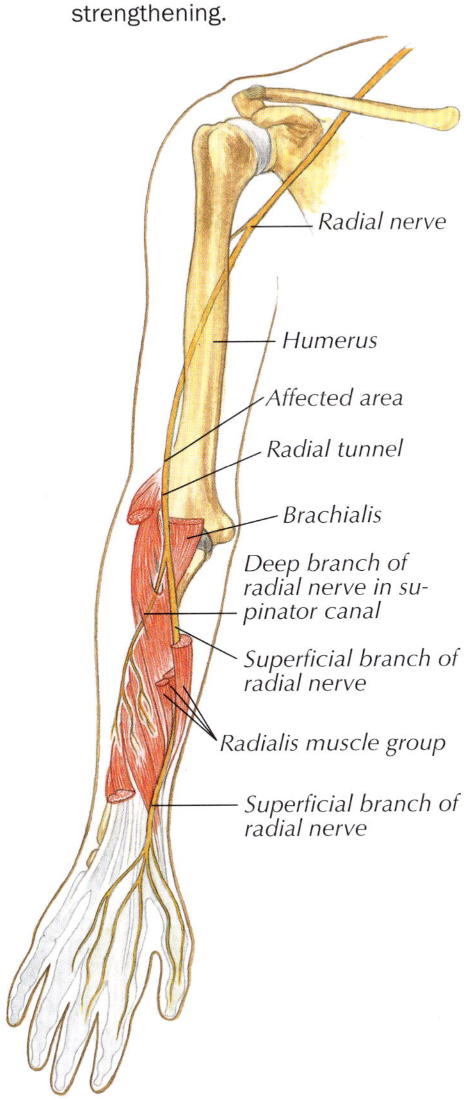

RECOVERY TIME WITH APPROPRIATE RECOVERY MANAGEMENT
4 to 6 weeks

Exercises

Stretching

- A gradual and pain-free increase in range of motion of the wrist and elbow joints.
- The radial nerve should be mobilized (flossed).
- Any tight muscles around neck, shoulders, upper back and upper torso. These muscles will differ from person to person.

Strengthening

- Strengthen any weak muscles around the neck, shoulders and upper back. These muscles will differ from person to person.
- The forearm extensors, supinators and pronators should be strengthened isometrically, concentrically and eccentrically.

See exercises
- *Radial nerve mobilization (page 102)*
- *Wrist extensors (page 140)*
- *Single-arm cable push (page 132)*

TENNIS ELBOW

Description

Tennis elbow is a painful condition of the wrist extensor tendons as they attach to the lateral epicondyle of the humerus. It is believed that repetitive over-use of the arm causes micro-trauma to the common extensor tendon over time. Direct trauma to the lateral epicondyle and entrapment of the radial nerve may also be potential causes. Despite the name, it isn't a common injury among tennis players and can affect almost any sport. It is more common in the over-30s age group.

Symptoms

- Pain around the lateral epicondyle region.
- Wrist extension and gripping movements will usually cause pain.

Causes

- Repetitive overuse of the arm.
- Rapid deceleration of the wrist during over-head sports such as tennis.
- Direct trauma to the lateral epicondyle of the humerus.
- Radial nerve adhering to the elbow joint capsule.

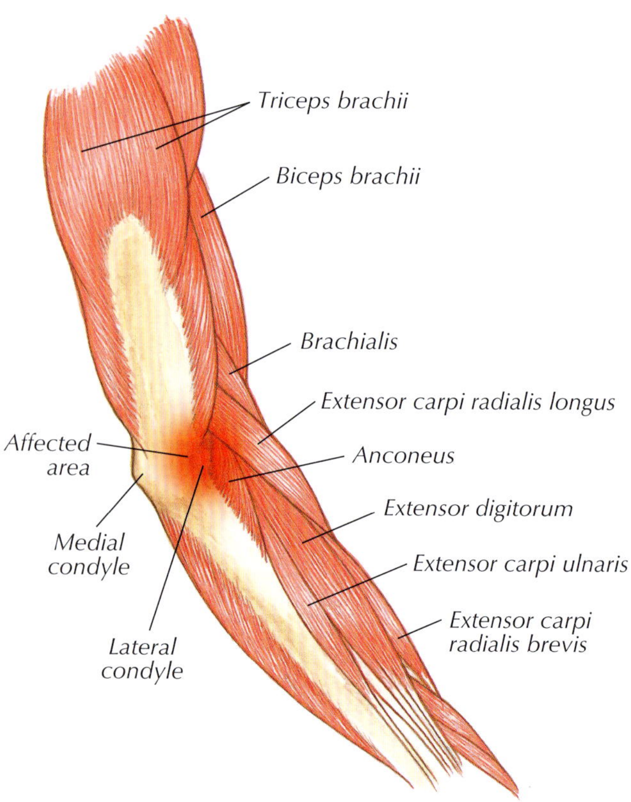

Treatment

Acute

- Rest from normal activities/training.
- Ice in the first 24 to 48 hours.
- Anti-inflammatory protocols.

Post-acute

- Heat therapy.
- Sports massage.
- Active Release Technique®.
- Gradual increase in range of motion of the wrist and elbow within pain-free ranges.
- Corrective exercise, especially improving muscle balance in the upper body, leading to gradual return to training (end-stage rehab) and competition to prevent re-injury.
- Strength training normally begins with isometric, then concentric and finally eccentric work is added.

RECOVERY TIME WITH APPROPRIATE RECOVERY MANAGEMENT
3 weeks to 3 months

Exercises

Stretching

- A gradual and pain-free increase in range of motion of the wrist and elbow joints.
- Any tight muscles around neck, shoulders, upper back and upper torso. These muscles will differ from person to person.

Strengthening

- Strengthen any weak muscles around the neck, shoulders and upper back. These muscles will differ from person to person.
- The forearm extensors should be strengthened isometrically, concentrically and eccentrically.

See exercises
- *Wrist extensors (page 140)*
- *Medicine ball shoulder external rotators (page 129)*

WRIST INJURIES

FRACTURED SCAPHOID

Description

The scaphoid is a peanut-shaped bone located on the thumb side, distal to the styloid process of the radius. It is one of eight carpal bones in the wrist and is the most commonly fractured bone in the wrist, often caused by breaking a fall with the hand. Sports that involve falls, such as skateboarding, cycling, BMX, snowboarding, downhill skiing, speed skating and horse riding are more vulnerable to this fracture.

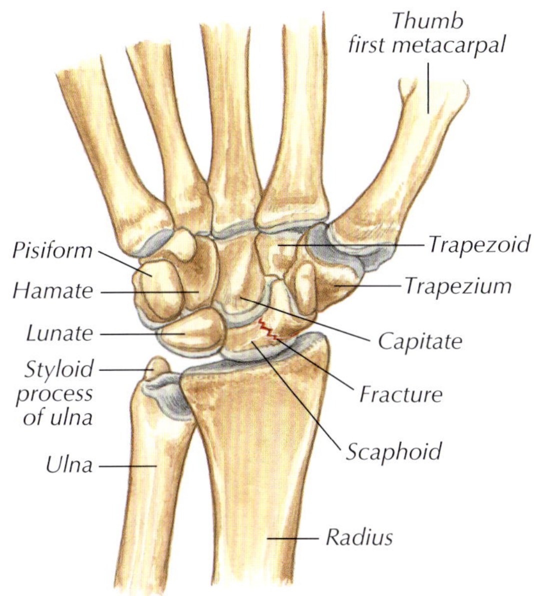

Symptoms

- Pain in the wrist.
- Pain and tenderness just below the thumb.
- Possible swelling at the site of the fracture.

Causes

- Breaking a fall with an outstretched hand.
- Direct trauma.

Treatment

- Wearing a cast for 9 to 12 weeks.
- An electrical stimulator may be used if the bone doesn't heal in the cast.
- Surgery may be used in some cases.
- Once the cast is removed, gradually increase the range of motion of the wrist within pain-free ranges.
- Strength training normally begins with isometric, then concentric and finally eccentric work is added. The forearm muscles will require strengthening.

RECOVERY TIME WITH APPROPRIATE RECOVERY MANAGEMENT
9 to 12 weeks (without surgery)
6 to 8 weeks (following surgery)

Exercises

Stretching

- A gradual and pain-free increase in range of motion of the wrist and elbow joints.

Strengthening

- The forearm flexors, extensors, supinators and pronators should be strengthened isometrically, concentrically and eccentrically.

See exercises
- *Wrist flexors (page 140)*
- *Wrist extensors (page 140)*

CARPAL TUNNEL SYNDROME

Description

This syndrome is a painful condition caused by entrapment or compression of the median nerve as it passes through the carpal tunnel, an opening through the wrist to the hand that is formed by the wrist bones on one side and the transverse carpal ligament on the other. This opening forms the carpal tunnel through which the median nerve and nine flexor tendons pass. Women are three times more likely than men to develop carpal tunnel syndrome. This is believed to be due to the smaller carpal tunnel in females.

Symptoms

- Numbness, tingling and burning in the thumb and fingers, especially the index and middle finger.
- Possible atrophy of the thenar eminence.
- Possible loss of grip strength.
- Pain can also develop in the arm and shoulder and swelling of the hand, which worsens at night.

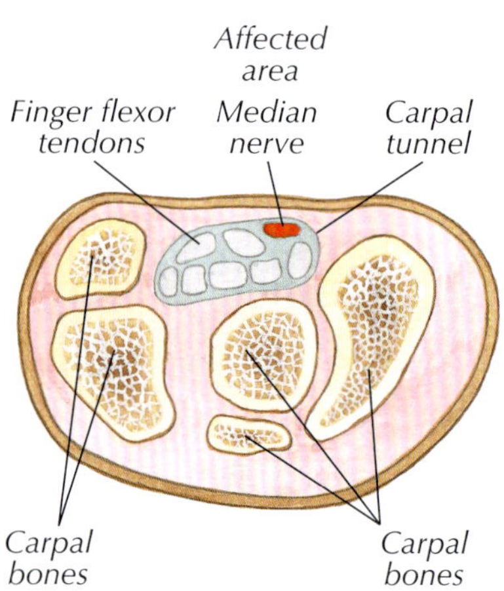

Cross-section of wrist

Causes

- Muscular, tendon or ligamentous inflammation.
- Abnormal bone growths, tumours and other space-occupying lesions.
- Obesity.
- Arthritis.
- Direct trauma to the area.
- Diabetes.

Treatment

Acute

- Rest from activities that exacerbate the condition.
- Ice therapy.
- Anti-inflammatory protocols.
- Splinting the wrist in some instances.

Post-acute

- Sports massage.
- Active Release Technique®.
- Gradual increase in range of motion of the wrist and elbow within pain-free ranges.
- Corrective exercise, especially improving muscle balance in the upper body, leading to gradual return to training (end-stage rehab) and competition to prevent re-injury.
- Strength training normally begins with isometric, then concentric and finally eccentric work is added. The forearm muscles may need strengthening.
- May need surgery in extreme cases to release the transverse carpal ligament.

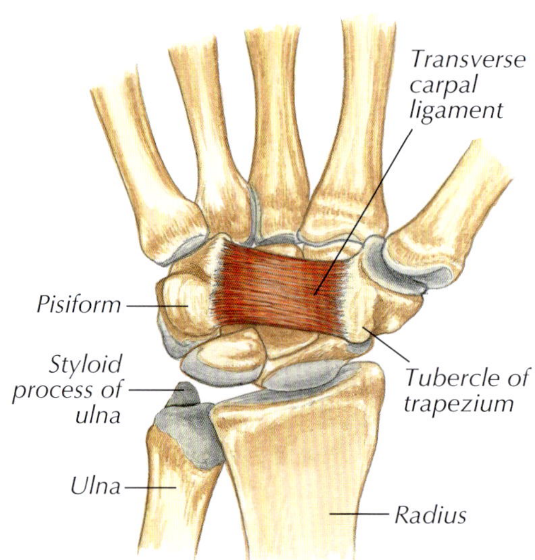

RECOVERY TIME WITH APPROPRIATE RECOVERY MANAGEMENT
4 to 6 weeks (without surgery)
Several months (after surgery)

Exercises

Stretching

- A gradual and pain-free increase in range of motion of the wrist and elbow joints.
- Any tight muscles around neck, shoulders, upper back and upper torso. These muscles will differ from person to person.

Strengthening

- Strengthen any weak muscles around the neck, shoulders and upper back. These muscles will differ from person to person.
- The forearm flexors, extensors, supinators and pronators should be strengthened isometrically, concentrically and eccentrically.

See exercises
- *Wrist flexors (page 140)*
- *Wrists extensors (page 140)*
- *Prone cobra (page 114)*

ENVIRONMENTAL INJURIES

DEHYDRATION

Description

Dehydration is an excessive loss of water from the body and occurs when the amount of water consumed is less than the amount used. Athletes who compete in vigorous, prolonged events in warm climates, such as triathletes, marathon runners, ultra distance runners, cricketers, cyclists are particularly vulnerable especially if they are unable to stop to take on fluids.

Symptoms

- Dry mouth.
- Lack of sweating.
- Lightheadedness.
- Muscle cramps.
- Nausea and vomiting.
- Heart palpitation.

Causes

- Excessive sweating; exercising in hot, humid, sunny conditions.
- Vomiting.
- Diarrhoea.
- Inability to take on fluids.

Treatment

- Small frequent intake of fluids.
- Fluids such as mineral water and/or electrolyte drinks should be used.
- A minimum intake of 0.033 litres of water per kilogram of body weight should be consumed on a daily basis.
- Caffeinated and overly sugary fluids should be avoided.
- Intravenous fluids may be required in extreme circumstances.

RECOVERY TIME WITH APPROPRIATE RECOVERY MANAGEMENT

A few hours to a few days

Exercises

- None

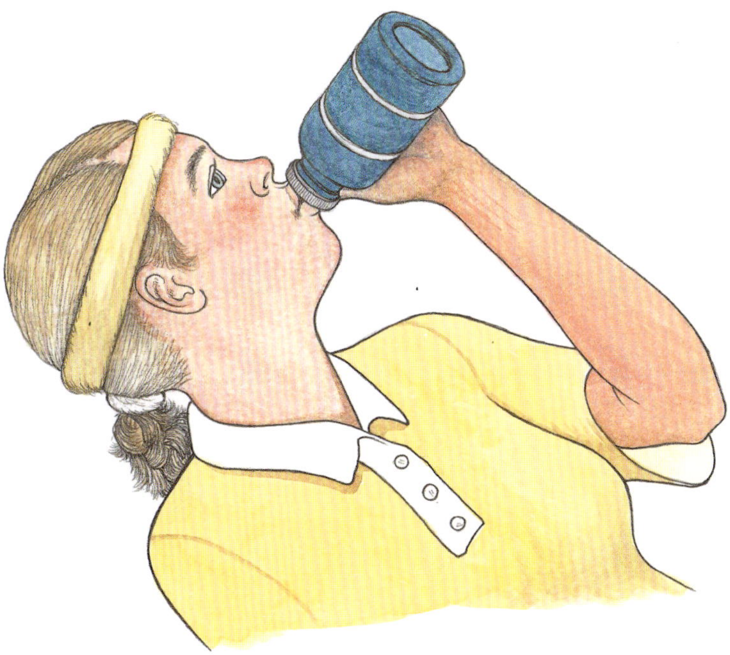

HEAT STROKE

Description

This is a potentially life-threatening condition where the body temperature is abnormally high with accompanying physiological and neurological symptoms. Heat stroke normally occurs in conditions of extreme heat, humidity and/or vigorous exercise in direct sunshine. Children and the elderly are most vulnerable due to their lower ability to control body temperature. Athletes who compete in vigorous, prolonged events in warm climates, such as triathletes, marathon runners, ultra-distance runners, cricketers, beach volleyball, cyclists and tennis players are also vulnerable.

Symptoms

- High body temperature.
- Absence of sweating, with hot red or flushed dry skin.
- Rapid pulse.
- Difficulty breathing.
- Strange behaviour.
- Hallucinations.
- Confusion.
- Agitation.
- Disorientation.
- Seizure.
- Possible coma.

Causes

- Exercising in extreme heat.
- Exercising in high humidity.
- Prolonged exercise in direct sunlight.
- Dehydration.

Treatment

- Seek immediate emergency medical treatment.
- Remove athlete to cool and shaded environment.
- Apply cool water to the skin.
- Fan the athlete with cool air.
- Place ice in the armpits and groin.

RECOVERY TIME WITH APPROPRIATE RECOVERY MANAGEMENT
A few days

Exercises

- None

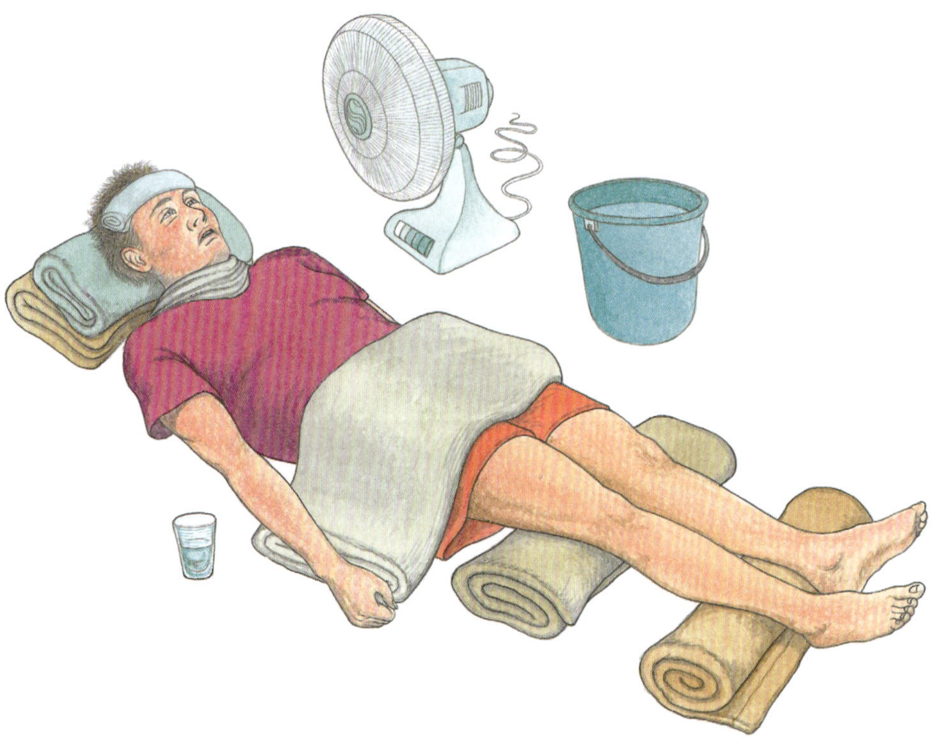

FROSTBITE

Description

Frostbite occurs when the affected areas of the body freeze. It occurs due to a lack of blood flow (and therefore heat) to the area and damaging ice crystals form. The most commonly affected areas are the hands, feet, nose and ears. Superficial frostbite affects the skin and subcutaneous tissues, while deep frostbite also affects muscle, tendons, nerves and bone. First-degree frostbite irritates the skin, second-degree frostbite causes blisters, but no major damage, while third-degree frostbite affects all skin layers and causes permanent tissue damage. Athletes who compete in events in cold climates are particularly vulnerable to frostbite and include mountaineers, cross-country skiers and bi-athletes. Children and the elderly are particularly vulnerable too.

Symptoms

- Pain, burning and numbness.
- Loss of sensation.
- The area may appear pale, red, blue or black depending on the severity.
- Clear or purplish blisters may appear.
- The affected area may feel hard to the touch.

Causes

- Exposure to extreme cold weather conditions.
- Lack of adequate clothing for the conditions.

Treatment

- Seek medical help as soon as possible.
- Remove the person from the cold conditions.
- Rewarm the affected area with moist heat (water at 40°C/104°F) for 15 to 30 minutes or until the area is thawed. If no thermometer is available, test the temperature with an unaffected hand to avoid burning the area. Beware, extreme pain may be felt as the area is rewarmed.
- Pain relief may be used.
- Dry heat should not be used as it can cause burning and dry out the injured tissue.
- The affected area should not be warmed if there is a risk of refreezing.
- Any blisters and wounds should be kept clean and dry. Aloe vera gel can be applied carefully.
- In extreme circumstances, amputation of the affected area is required.

RECOVERY TIME WITH APPROPRIATE RECOVERY MANAGEMENT
A few weeks to several months

Exercises

- None

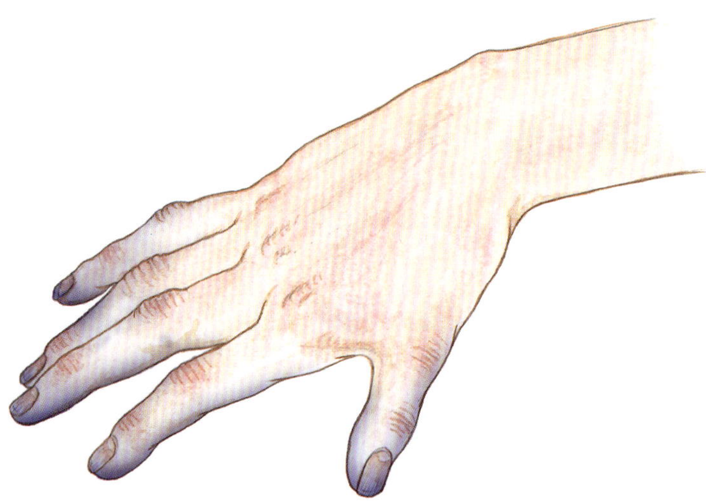

HYPOTHERMIA

Description

Hypothermia is a reduction in body temperature to below 35 °C (95 °F). Hypothermia is a potentially life-threatening condition due to the risk of organ failure. It is normally caused by exposure to cold conditions, inadequate warm clothing and/or immersion in water (including exposure to rain). Athletes who compete in events in cold or wet climates, such as mountaineers, cross-country skiers, sailors, water skiers and surfers are particularly vulnerable. Children and the elderly are particularly vulnerable too.

Symptoms

- Initially a sensation of feeling cold, often accompanied with shivering.
- Initial hunger and nausea, giving way to apathy.
- Confusion.
- Lethargy.
- Slurred speech.
- Loss of consciousness.
- Coma.

Causes

- Exposure to extreme cold weather conditions.
- Exposure to wet conditions.
- Lack of adequate clothing for the conditions.

Treatment

- Seek medical help as soon as possible.
- Remove the person from the cold conditions into a warm, sheltered area.
- Wet clothing should be removed and replaced with dry clothing, including on the head.
- Breathing should be monitored and CPR given if appropriate.
- Warm blankets and body-to-body contact should be used to rewarm the body.

RECOVERY TIME WITH APPROPRIATE RECOVERY MANAGEMENT
Minutes to a few hours

Exercises

- None

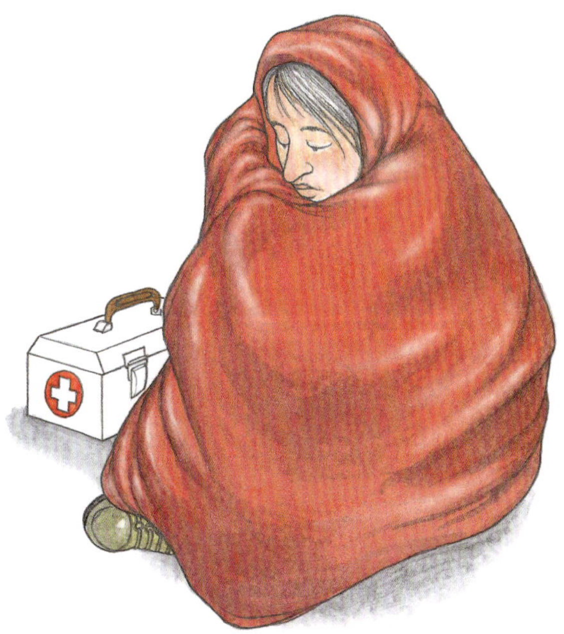

SUN BURN

Description

Sun burn is an inflammatory condition of the skin caused by overexposure to ultraviolet radiation from the sun. Athletes who compete in events in warm, sunny climates (especially between the hours of 10 am and 3 pm) are particularly vulnerable, including cricketers, cyclists, tennis players, beach volleyball players and track-and-field athletes. Water and snow-based sports, such as sailing, canoeing, rowing, skiing and snow boarding may also be vulnerable due to the reflection of sunlight off the water or the snow. High altitude and being close to the equator also increase the risk. Athletes with pale skin are more vulnerable than those with darker skin.

Symptoms

- Red, tender and hot skin.
- Pain with palpation or rubbing of the skin.
- Possible dehydration.
- Possible swelling, blistering and peeling of the skin.
- Possible skin rash.

Causes

- Time spent in direct sunlight, especially in summer months during the middle of the day.
- Exposing the skin to sunlight without using sun block and/or clothing to protect the skin. Melanocytes produce melanin to protect skin from UV rays. If UV rays exceed what can be blocked by the level of melanin, then the result is sunburn.

Treatment

- Remove the person from direct sunlight into the shade.
- If there is no shade available, cover up with clothing.
- Drink cool water if the sun burn is not severe.
- Apply cool damp compresses over the affected areas.
- Soak in a cool bath – dry off by dabbing with a towel (not rubbing).
- Apply aloe vera gel over affected areas.
- Clean bandages should be applied to any blistered areas.
- Seek medical help if the symptoms are severe.

RECOVERY TIME WITH APPROPRIATE RECOVERY MANAGEMENT
2 to 7 days

Exercises

- None

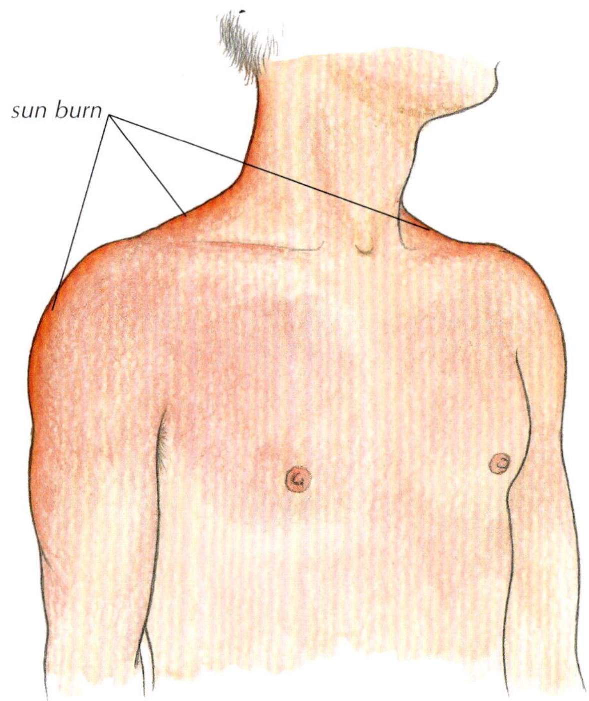

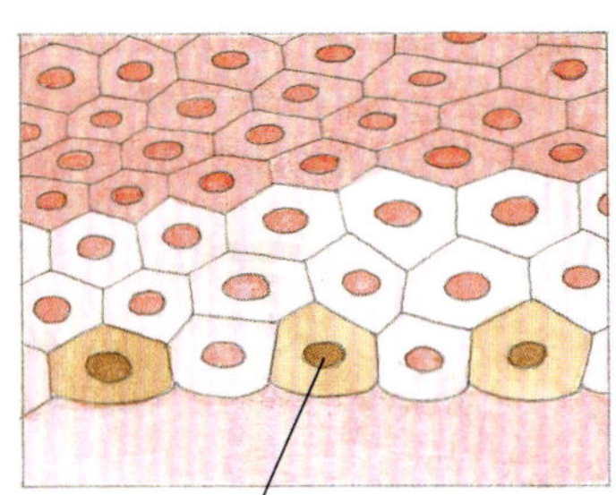

PART 3 – REHABILITATION

MOBILIZATIONS

MCKENZIE PUSH-UP

Basic description:

- Inhale, then as you exhale, push through the arms, raising each vertebra one at a time from the top towards the bottom.
- Keep the front pelvic bones (anterior superior iliac spines) in contact with the ground.
- Go as far as you can without the pelvic bones leaving the floor and return to the start position while inhaling.
- Try to move further each time with good form.

Tips for good form:

- Keep your pelvic bones in contact with the ground
- Keep your head in line with the spine (do not flex or extend your head or neck).

Note: *If you experience pain doing this mobilization do not continue performing it and seek professional advice.*

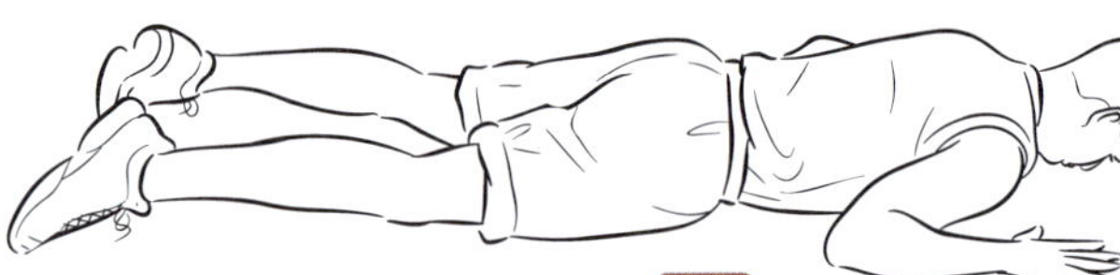

STARTING POSITION

- Lie face down (prone), elbows bent and palms down (pronated) next to your shoulders.

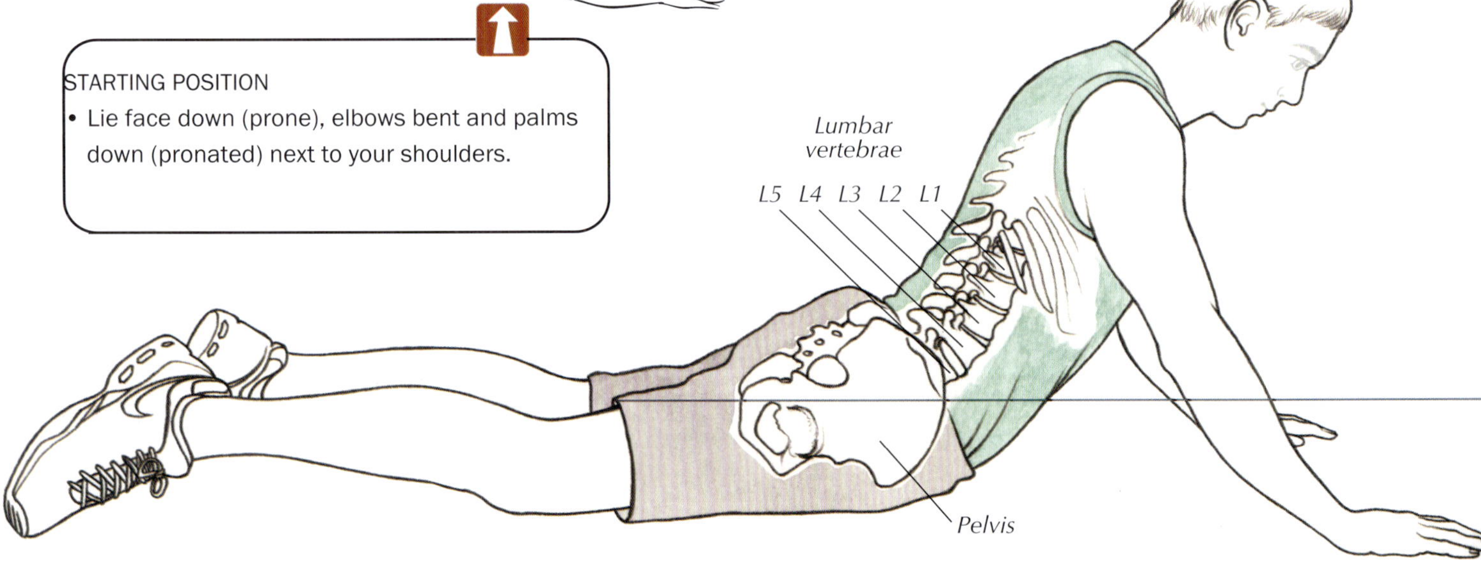

ANALYSIS OF MOVEMENT–L5	*REGION*	*JOINT MOVEMENT*	*JOINTS*
Joint 1	Lumbar spine	Up: extension	L1

MEDIAN NERVE MOBILIZATION

Basic description:

- Bend your head sideways until you feel a stretch in the nerve and then allow some slack on the nerve by bringing the head back towards the middle a little.
- Keeping a continuous tension on the nerve, flex the wrist as you side-bend the head away, then extend the wrist as you bring your head back towards the middle.

Tips for good form:

- Do not do this too aggressively. You should not have any pain or pins and needles in the arm, neck or shoulder.

STARTING POSITION

- Stand with the target arm away from your body.
- Externally rotate your shoulder and fully extend your elbow and wrist.

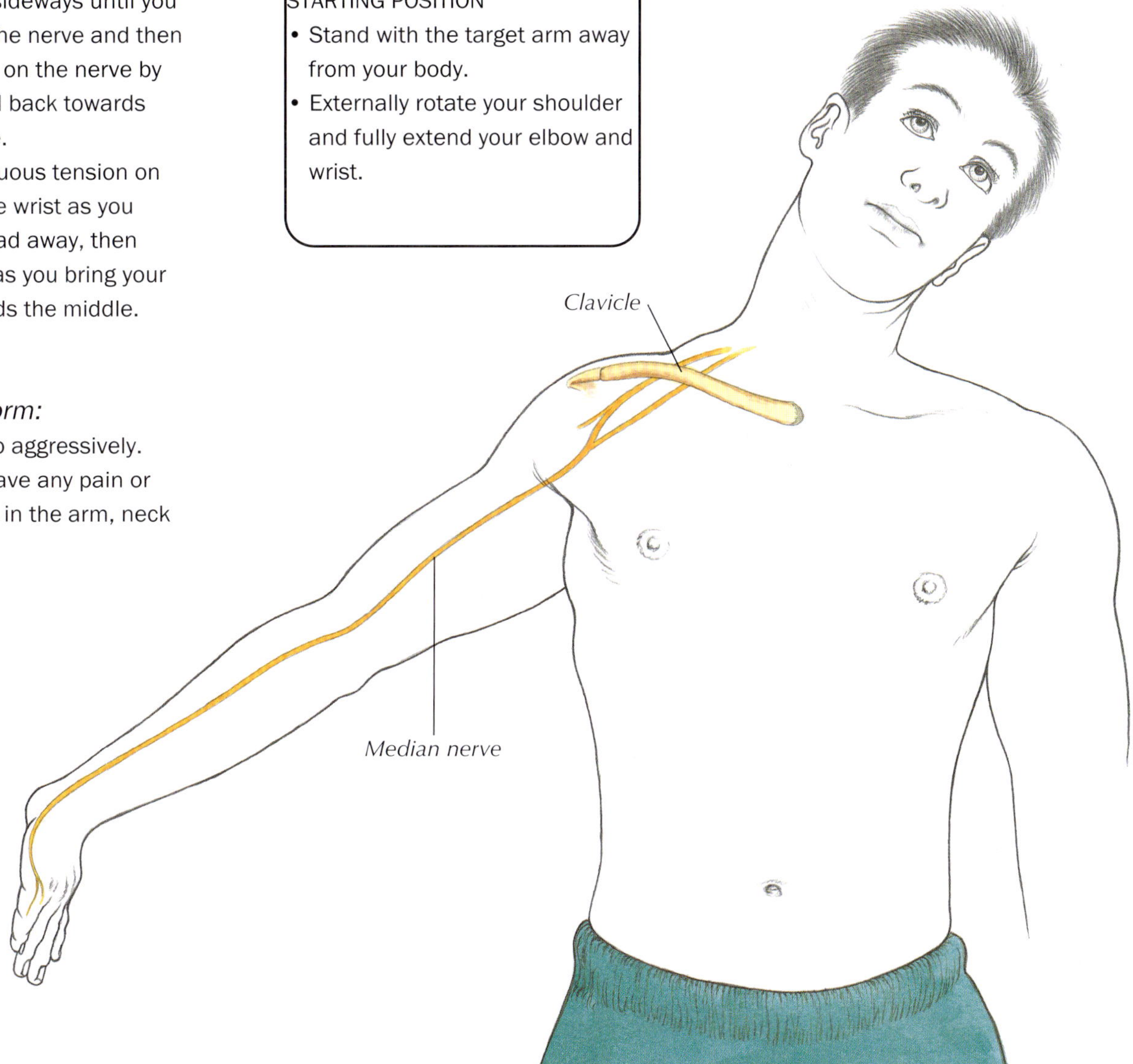

*ANALYSIS OF MOVEMENT*Median	*REGION*	*JOINT MOVEMENT*	*NERVE*
Joint 1	Neck	Side flexion	Median
Joint 2	Shoulder	Abduction, external rotation	Median
Joint 3	Elbow	Extension	Median
Joint 4	Wrist	Extension, flexion	

RADIAL NERVE MOBILIZATION

Basic description:

- Bend your head sideways until you feel a stretch in the nerve, abduct the shoulder, then allow some slack on the nerve by bringing the head back towards the middle a little.
- Keeping a continuous tension on the nerve, extend the wrist as you side-bend the head away, then flex the wrist as you bring the head back towards the middle.

STARTING POSITION

- Stand with the target arm away from your body.
- Internally rotate the shoulder and fully flex the thumb, fingers and wrist with the elbow fully extended.

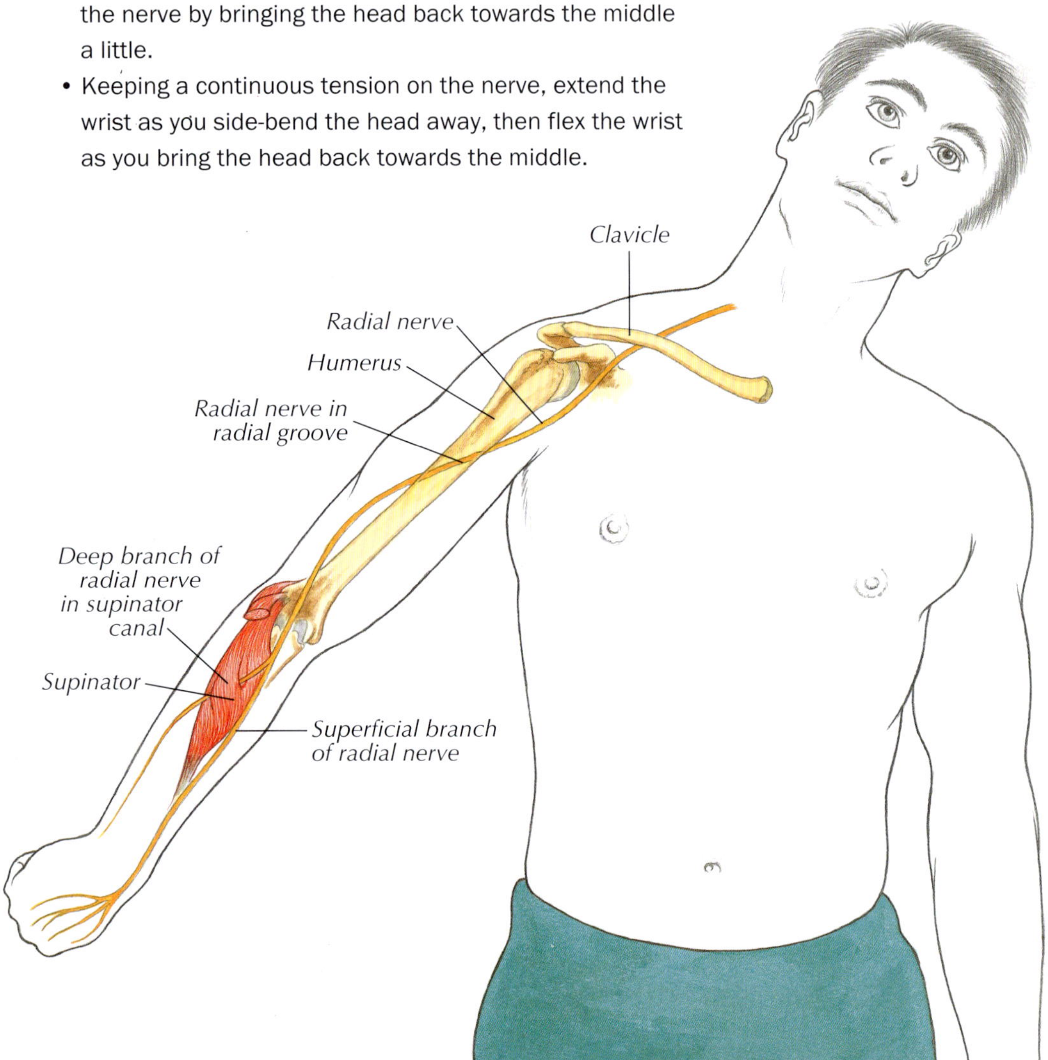

Tips for good form:

- Do not do this too aggressively. You should not have any pain or pins and needles in the arm, neck or shoulder.

*ANALYSIS OF MOVEMENT*Radial	*REGION*	*JOINT MOVEMENT*	*NERVE*
Joint 1	Neck	Side flexion	Radial
Joint 2	Shoulder	Abduction, internal rotation	Radial
Joint 3	Elbow	Extension	Radial
Joint 4	Wrist	Flexion, extension	

SHOULDER MOBILIZATIONS

STARTING POSITION
- Stand with the target arm by your side.

Basic description:
- Move the shoulder joint (lift the arm) into pain-free ranges in all planes.
- Move the arm forwards, backwards, up and down and out to the side as far as you can without pain.

Tips for good form:
- Maintain good posture throughout.
- Do not do this too aggressively as to cause pain or muscle spasm.

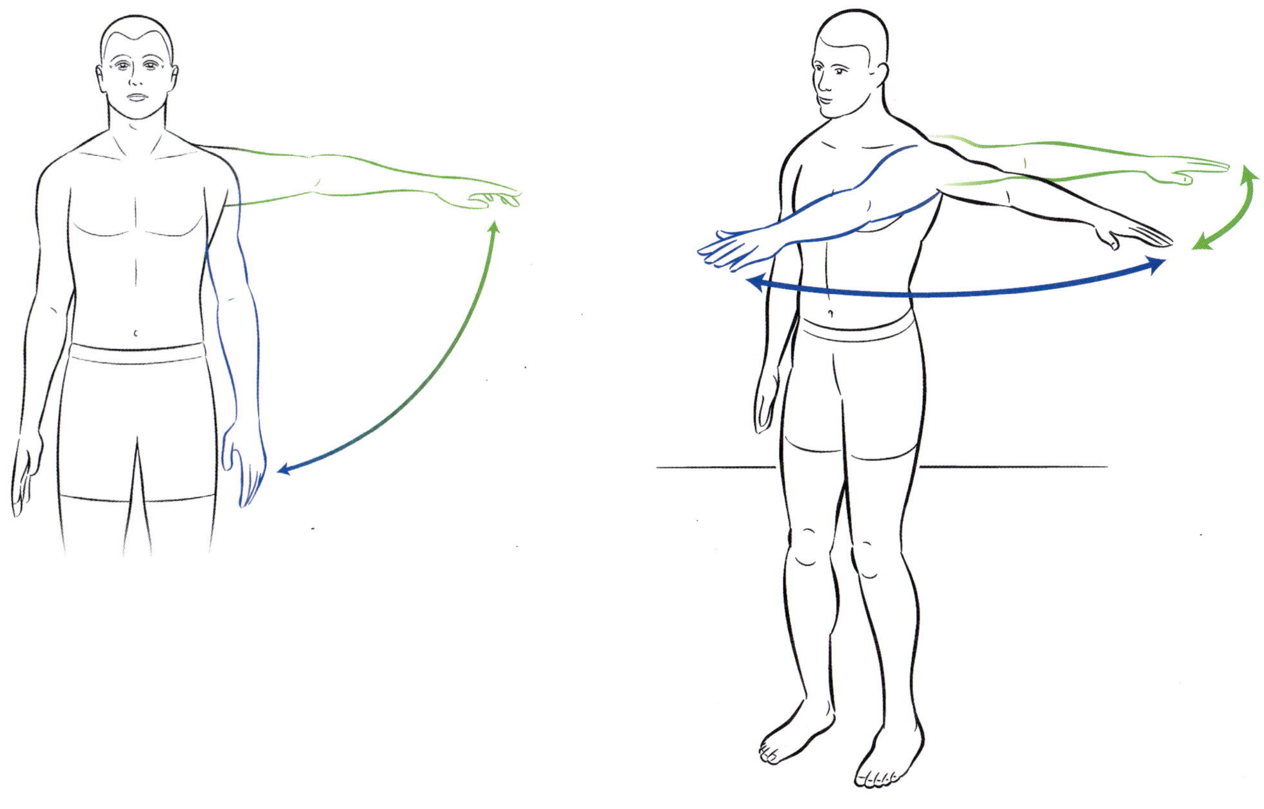

ANALYSIS OF MOVEMENT- pula	*JOINTS*	*JOINT MOVEMENT*	*MOBILIZING MUSCLES*
Joint 1	Shoulder	Flexion, extension, abduction, internal rotation, external rotation	Deltoid, pectoralis major, biceps brachii, coracobrachialis, latissimus dorsi, teres major, infraspinatus, teres minor, triceps brachii (fibres of long head), supraspinatus, subscapularis
Joint 2	Shoulder girdle (scapula)	Abduction, adduction, upward and downward rotation	Trapezius, rhomboids, serratus anterior, pectoralis minor, levator sca

STRETCHES

ABDOMINALS

Basic description:

- To increase the stretch, extend the knees allowing your head to move further towards the floor until you feel a stretch in your abdominals.
- Breathe in and out through your nose, allowing your abdomen to rise and fall with each breath. Every two or three breaths, increase the stretch on the exhalation.
- Continue for one to two minutes.

STARTING POSITION

- Begin by lying supine (face up) over a Swiss ball, with your sacrum, spine and head all in contact with the ball and with knees bent.
- Place your arms overhead.

Note: *If you ever feel dizzy while looking upwards, for instance when looking in overhead cupboards or looking up at aeroplanes, DO NOT perform this stretch. If you feel faint or dizzy doing this stretch, stop immediately. You may wish to have your neck checked by a trained professional for vertebral artery occlusion.*

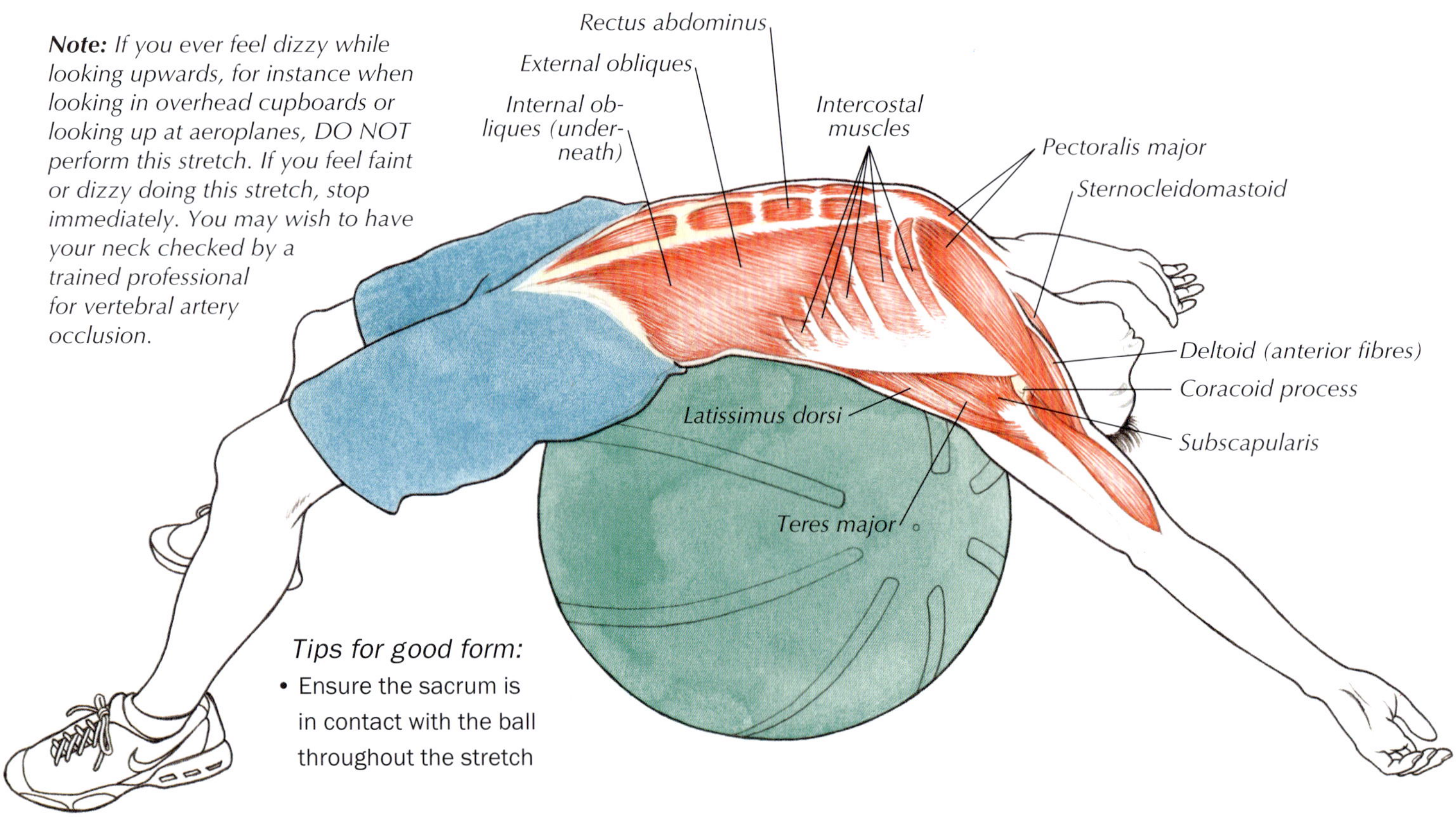

Tips for good form:

- Ensure the sacrum is in contact with the ball throughout the stretch

ANALYSIS OF MOVEMENT- major	*JOINTS*	*JOINT POSITION*	*MUSCLES STRETCHED*
Joint 1	Cervical spine	Extension	Sternocleidomastoid, scalenes (anterior fibres), longus capitis, longus coli
Joint 2	Thoracic and lumbar spine	Extension	Rectus abdominus, external obliques, internal obliques, internal intercostals, serratus posterior inferior
Joint 3	Shoulder	Flexion, abduction, external rotation	Pectoralis major, deltoid (anterior fibres), subscapularis, latissimus dorsi, teres

ADDUCTORS

Basic description:

- Increase the bend in the non-stretching leg, moving slightly forwards on the ball until you feel a stretch.
- Inhale and contract the foot of the leg that is being stretched into the floor for five seconds.
- Relax and, as you exhale, move further into the stretch by bending the opposite knee. Hold the new position for five seconds and repeat three to five times.

Tips for good form:

- Keep the knee of the non-stretching leg in line with the second toe.
- Keep the torso upright.
- Keep the whole foot of the leg being stretched in contact with the ground throughout.

STARTING POSITION

- Sit upright on a Swiss ball. Take the leg to be stretched out to the side, keeping the foot facing forwards.
- The other leg should be facing forwards at an approximate 45° angle, knees directly in line with the second toe.

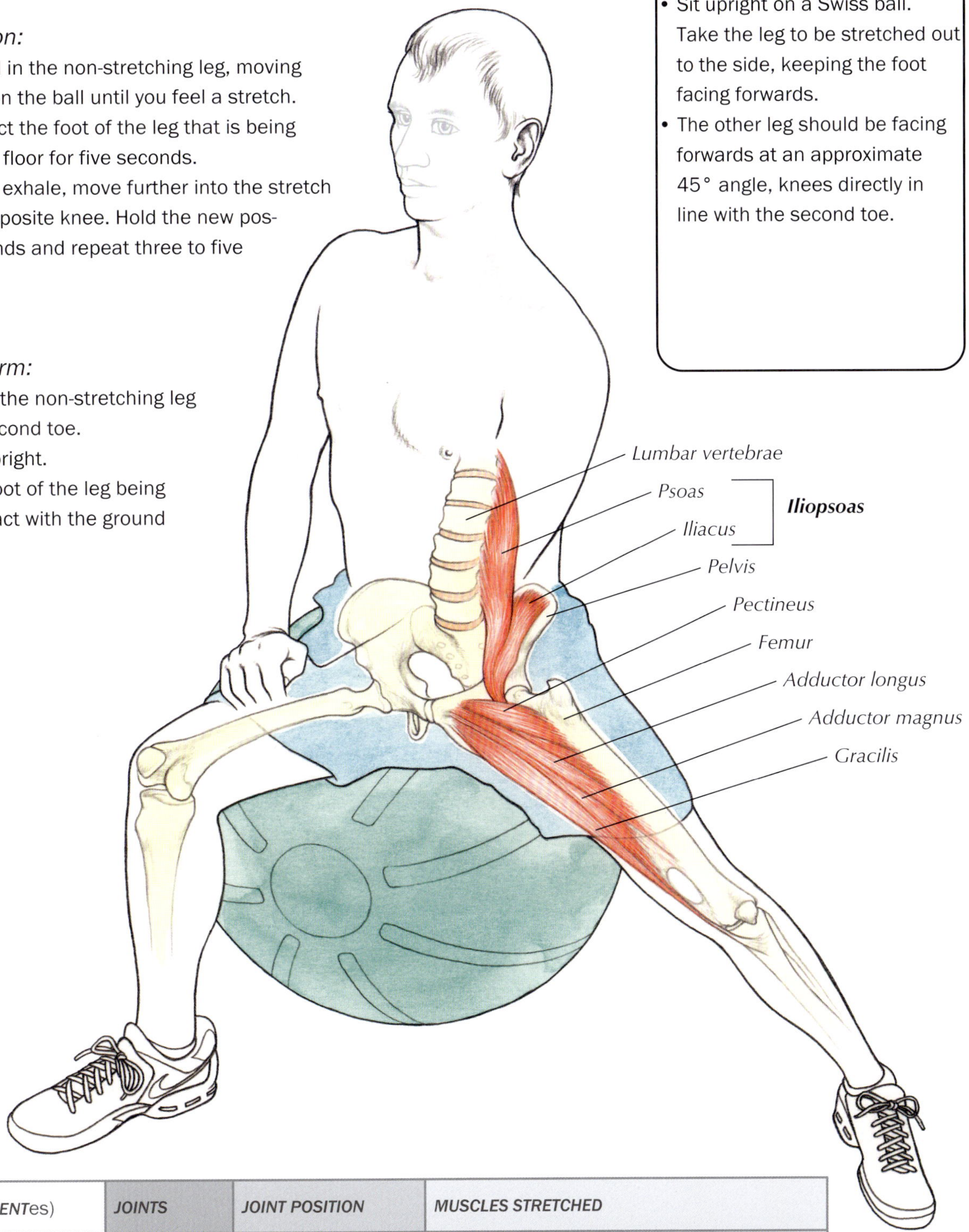

*ANALYSIS OF MOVEMENT*es)	*JOINTS*	*JOINT POSITION*	*MUSCLES STRETCHED*
Joint 1	Hip	Abduction	Pectineus, adductor brevis, adductor longus, adductor magnus, gracilis, psoas, iliacus, gluteus maximus (lower fibr

ANTERIOR TIBIALIS

Basic description:

- Plantarflex and evert the ankle on the lifted leg.
- Hold the stretch for 30 seconds or more while breathing naturally.
- Repeat three to five times or until no improvement is made.

Tips for good form:

- Maintain good posture throughout the body.

STARTING POSITION

- Begin standing with feet together. Lift the leg that requires the stretch.

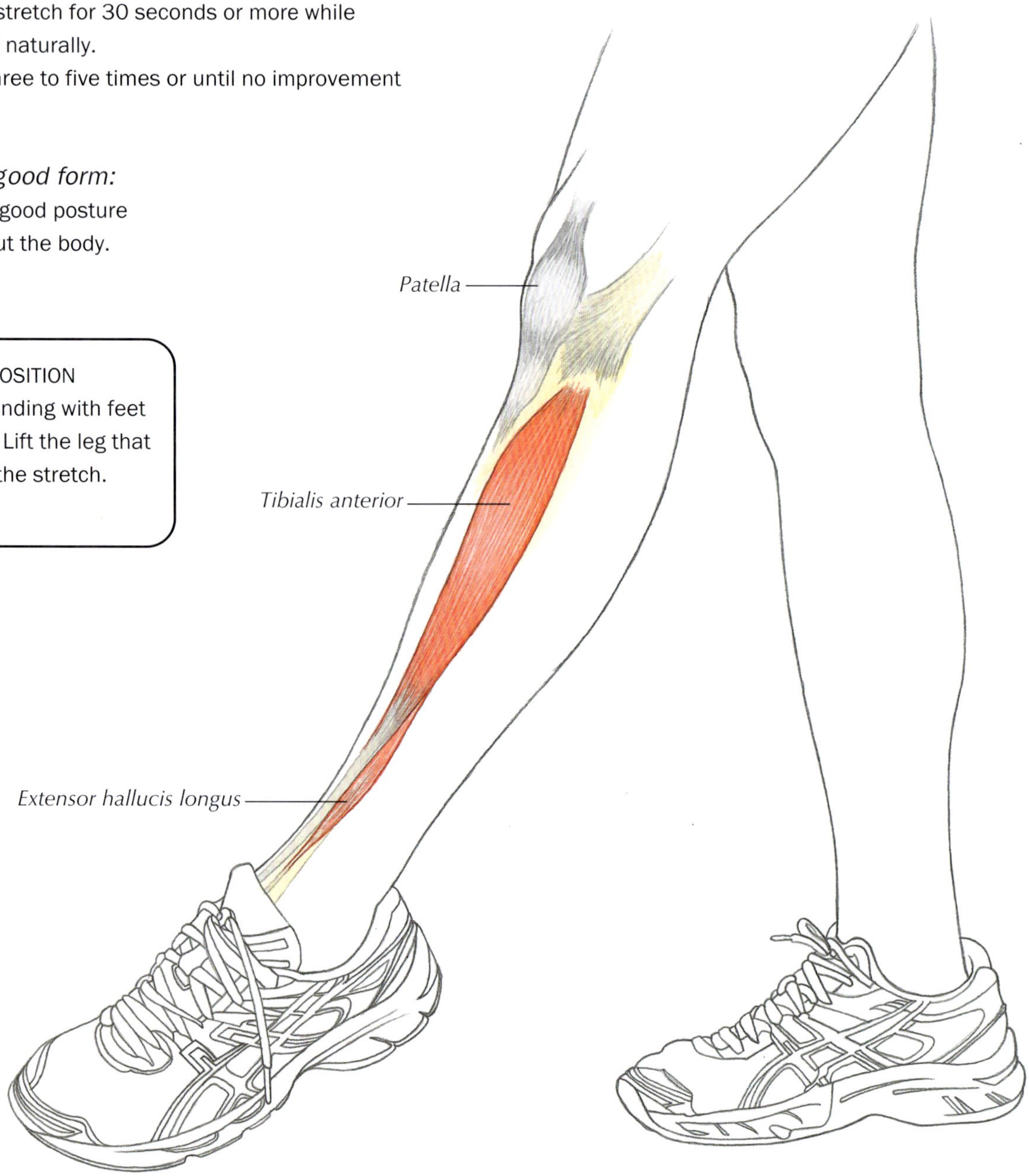

*ANALYSIS OF MOVEMENT*gus	*JOINTS*	*JOINT POSITION*	*MUSCLES STRETCHED*
Joint 1	Ankle	Plantarflexion, Eversion	Tibialis anterior, extensor hallucis lon

CALF STRETCH

Basic description:

- Lean your body weight towards the wall until you feel a stretch in the calf of the back leg.
- Inhale, then push the ball of the back foot into the ground for five seconds.
- Relax and as you exhale, lean further into the wall to increase the stretch until you reach a new position of 'bind'. Hold the new position for five seconds.
- Repeat three to five times or until no improvement is made.

Tips for good form:

- Keep the back foot perpendicular to the wall or turned in slightly.
- Keep the back knee straight.
- Keep good spinal alignment and chin tucked in.

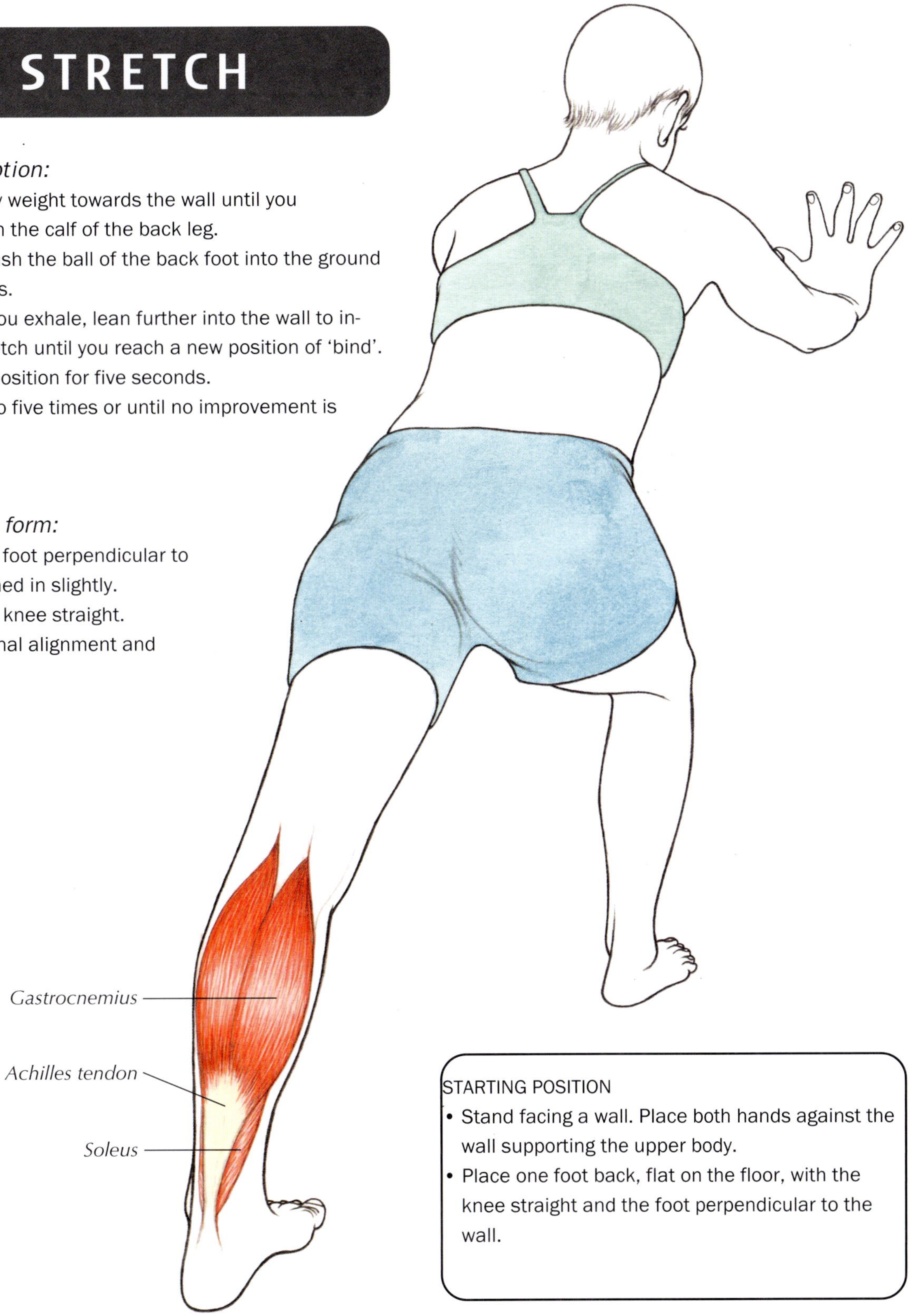

STARTING POSITION

- Stand facing a wall. Place both hands against the wall supporting the upper body.
- Place one foot back, flat on the floor, with the knee straight and the foot perpendicular to the wall.

*ANALYSIS OF MOVEMENT*vis	*JOINTS*	*JOINT POSITION*	*MUSCLES STRETCHED*
Joint 1	Hip	Dorsiflexion	Gastrocnemius, soleus, tibialis posterior, peroneus longus and bre

HAMSTRINGS – SEATED ON A SWISS BALL

Basic description:

- Keeping the pinched skin between your fingers, bend forwards from the hips until you feel a stretch in your hamstrings.
- Inhale, then pull your heels into the ground, contracting your hamstrings for five seconds.
- Relax, and as you exhale, lean further forwards from the hips to increase the stretch until you reach a new position of 'bind'. Hold the new position for five seconds.
- Repeat three to five times or until no improvement is made.

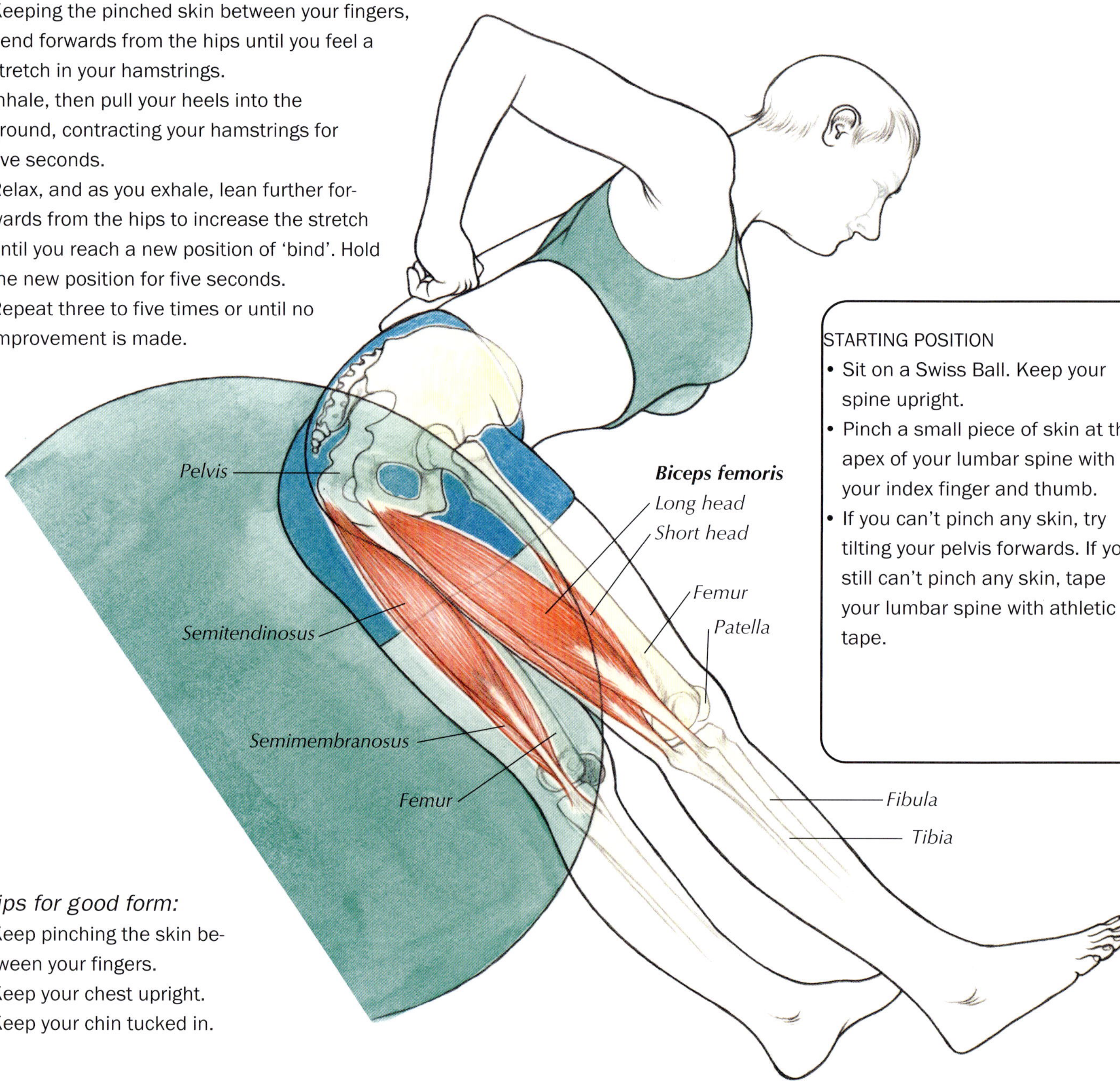

STARTING POSITION

- Sit on a Swiss Ball. Keep your spine upright.
- Pinch a small piece of skin at the apex of your lumbar spine with your index finger and thumb.
- If you can't pinch any skin, try tilting your pelvis forwards. If you still can't pinch any skin, tape your lumbar spine with athletic tape.

Tips for good form:

- Keep pinching the skin between your fingers.
- Keep your chest upright.
- Keep your chin tucked in.

*ANALYSIS OF MOVEMENT*sus	*JOINTS*	*JOINT POSITION*	*MUSCLES STRETCHED*
Joint 1	Hip	Flexion	Biceps femoris, semitendinosus, semimembrano

NECK EXTENSORS

STARTING POSITION
- Start seated or standing with good posture.
- One hand on chin/lower jaw.

Basic description:

- Tuck your chin in towards the neck. You can use one hand to push and hold the chin inwards.
- When you feel a stretch on the upper extensors on the back of the neck just below the back of the skull (occiput), place the other hand on the back of the head.

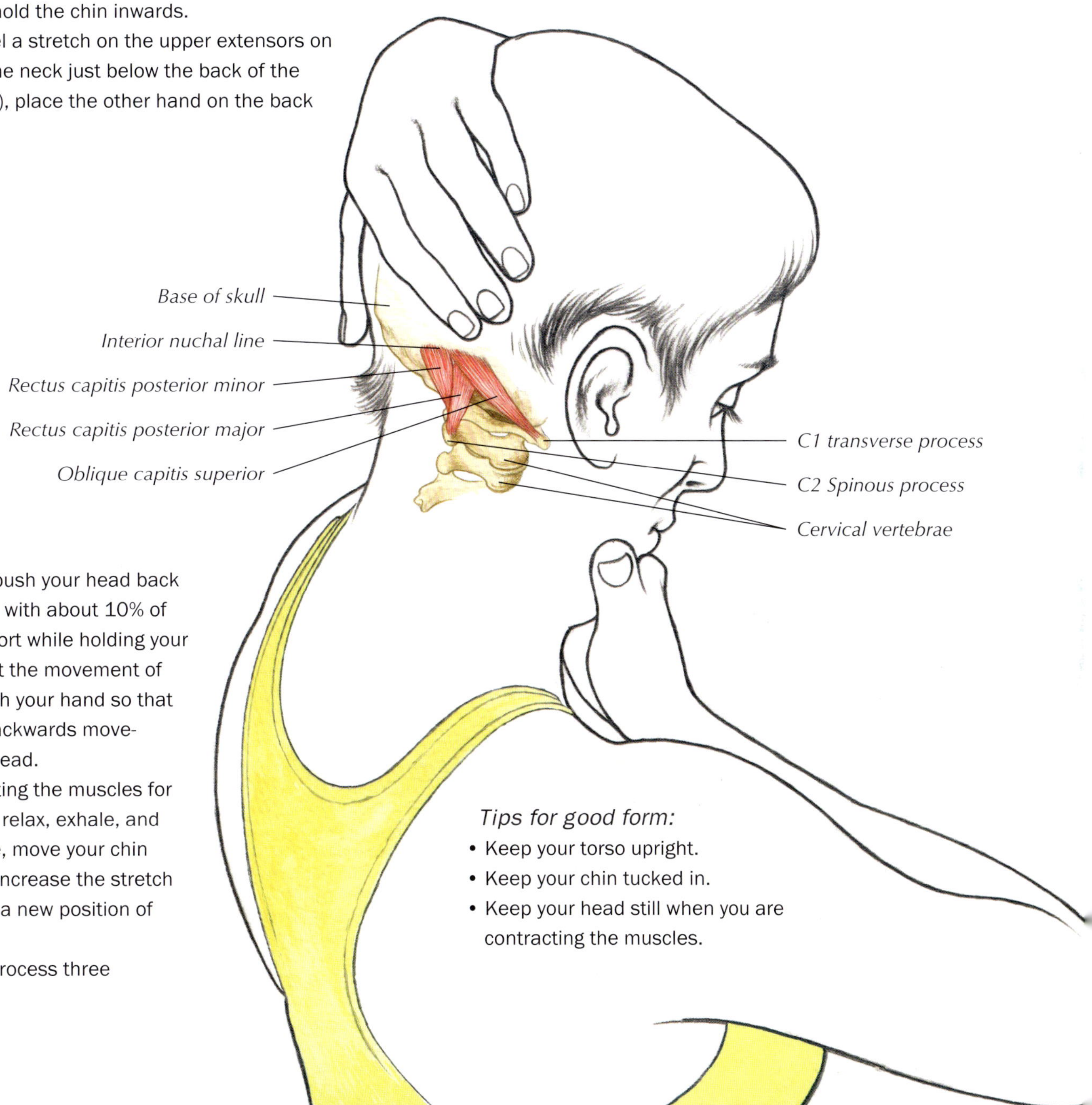

- Inhale, then push your head back into the hand with about 10% of maximum effort while holding your breath. Resist the movement of your head with your hand so that there is no backwards movement of the head.
- After contracting the muscles for five seconds, relax, exhale, and as you exhale, move your chin inwards and increase the stretch until you find a new position of 'bind'.
- Repeat this process three to five times.

Tips for good form:

- Keep your torso upright.
- Keep your chin tucked in.
- Keep your head still when you are contracting the muscles.

*ANALYSIS OF MOVEMENT*is.	*JOINTS*	*JOINT POSITION*	*MUSCLES STRETCHED*
Joint 1	Occipital/Atlas (C1–C3)	Flexion	Rectus capitis posterior major and minor, oblique capitis superior, semispinalis capit

PECTORALIS MINOR

Basic description:

- Allow your body weight to drop towards the floor keeping your shoulders parallel to the ground.
- When you feel a stretch just below your armpit (axilla), inhale and push your elbow and forearm into the ball with about 10% of maximum effort while holding your breath.
- After contracting the muscle for five seconds, relax, exhale and as you do so, move the torso further towards the floor until you find a new position of 'bind'.
- Repeat this process three to five times.

Tips for good form:

- Ensure that your shoulder is supported by the ball throughout the stretch.
- When increasing the stretch, allow the scapula (shoulder blade) to move towards the spine.

STARTING POSITION

- Start on all fours. Place one elbow on the apex of a Swiss ball.
- Support your shoulder on the ball.

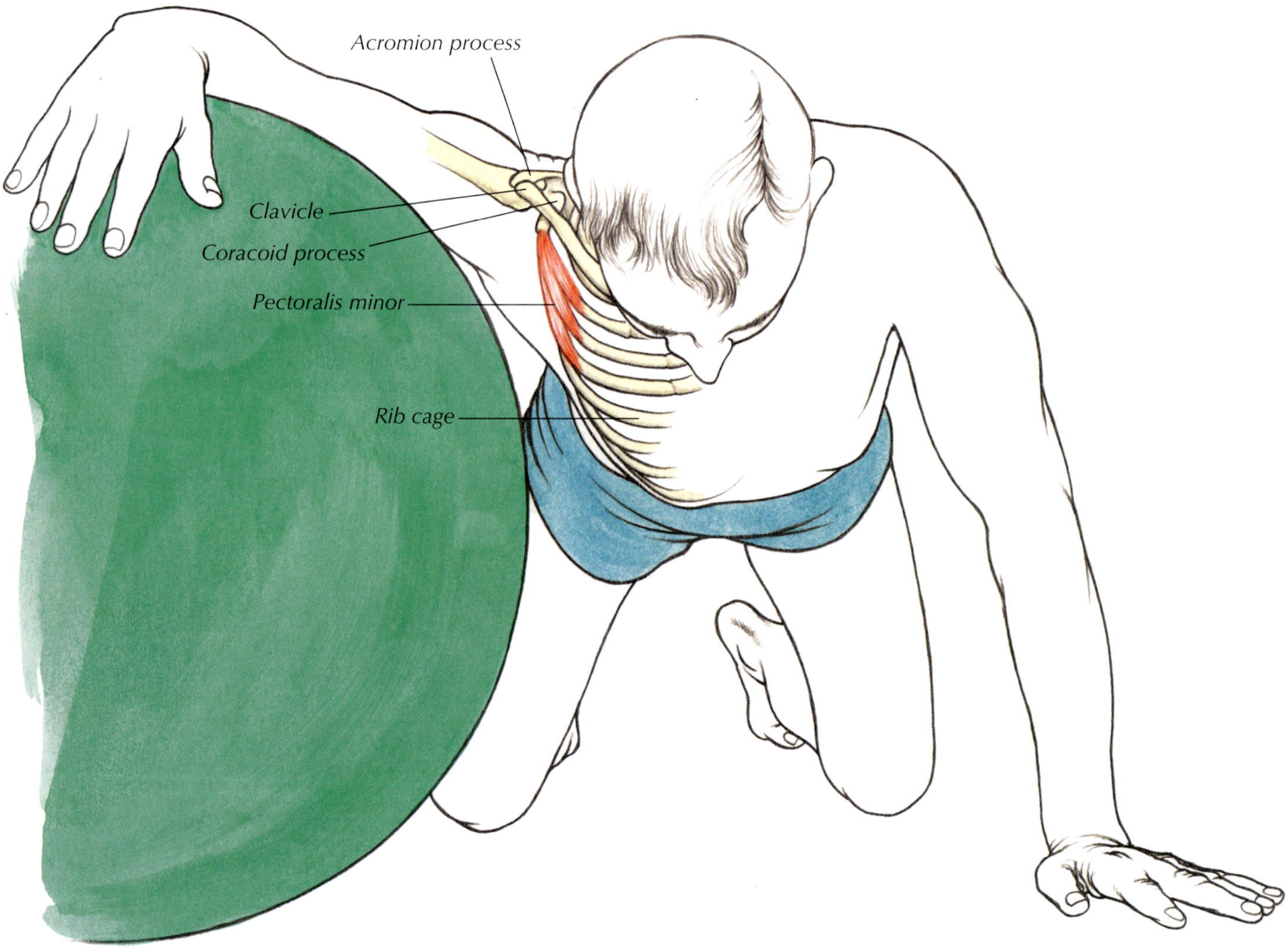

*ANALYSIS OF MOVEMENT*nor	*JOINTS*	*JOINT POSITION*	*JOINTS*
Joint 1	Scapulothoracic	Retraction	Pectoralis mi

QUADRICEPS

STARTING POSITION

- Kneel with one leg forwards, foot flat on the floor, and the other leg behind you. Rest your back shin against a Swiss ball, with the knee on the floor cushioned on an exercise mat or towel.
- Keep the torso upright.
- If balancing is a challenge, you may wish to reach back and support the ball with your hands.

Basic description:

- Posteriorly rotate your pelvis (tuck the pelvis under) to feel the stretch.
- Inhale, then push the shin into the ball for five seconds.
- Relax and as you exhale posteriorly, tuck your pelvis further under to increase the stretch until you reach a new position of 'bind'. Hold the new position for five seconds.
- Repeat three to five times or until no improvement is made.

Tips for good form:

- Keep good spinal alignment and your chin tucked in.
- If the stretch is too intense, move your knee away from the ball until it is comfortable.

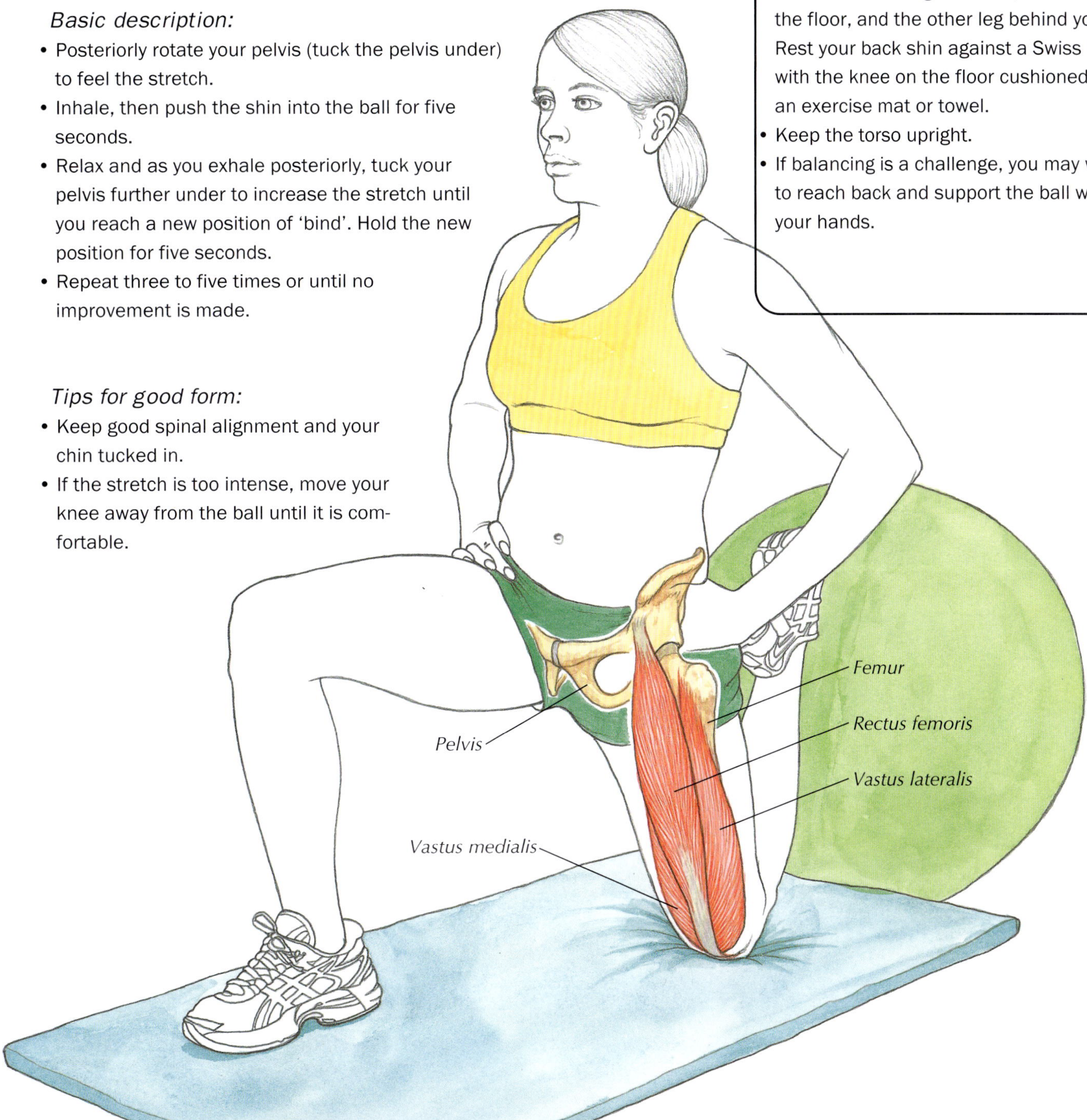

ANALYSIS OF MOVEMEN-Toris	JOINTS	JOINT POSITION	MUSCLES STRETCHED
Joint 1	Knee	Flexion	Vastus medialis, vastus intermedius, vastus lateralis, rectus femoris
Joint 2	Hip	Extension	Rectus fem

TENSOR FASCIA LATA

Basic description:

- Push your pelvis towards the wall while pushing downwards on the outer pelvis.
- Breathe slowly and deeply, and relax into the stretch. Hold the stretch for 30–60 seconds, easing into the stretch with every two or three exhalations.

Tips for good form:

- Ensure your pelvis furthest from the wall stays in line with the pelvis nearest to the wall.
- Keep your feet flat on the floor and parallel to the wall.

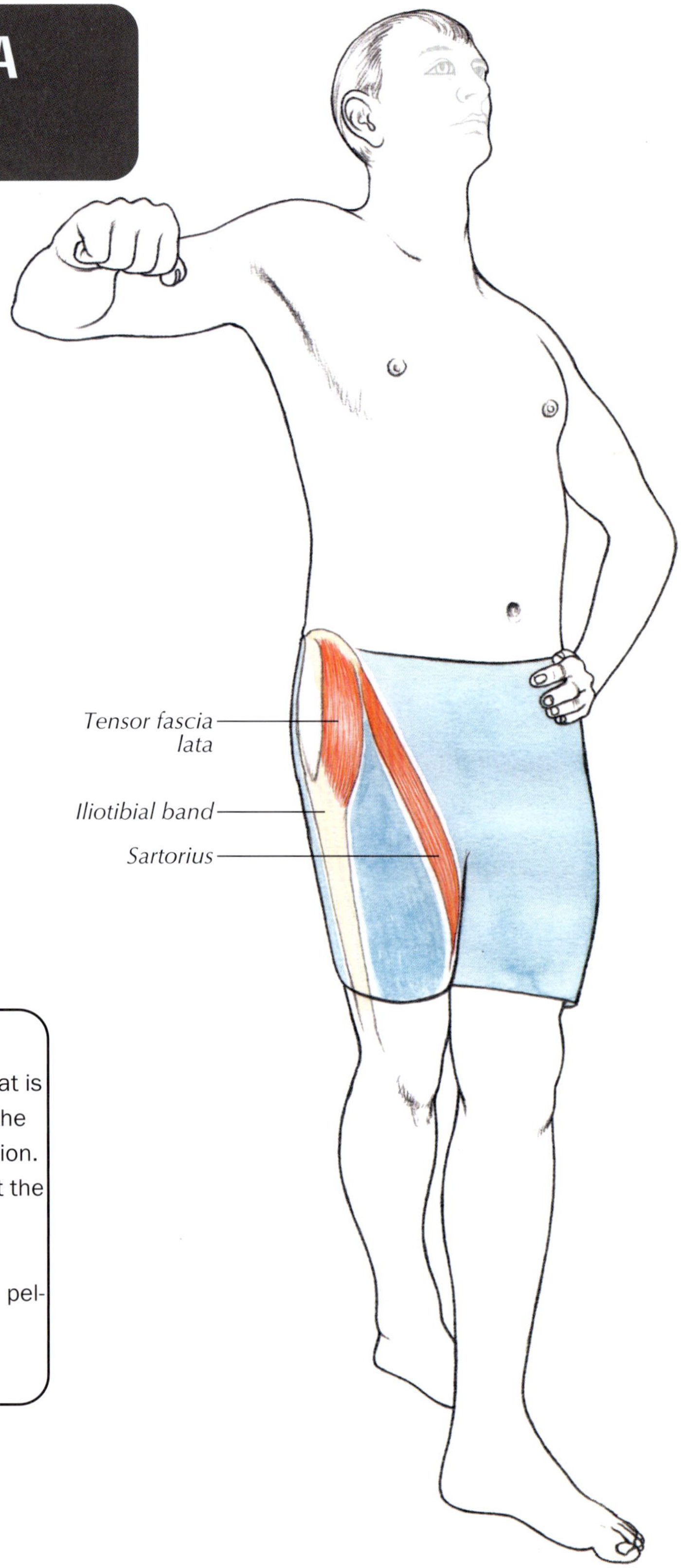

STARTING POSITION

- Stand side-on to a wall. The leg of the side that is to be stretched is placed across and behind the other leg so that it is in adduction and extension.
- Place your forearm closest to the wall against the wall, taking the weight of your torso.
- Place your hand furthest from the wall on the pelvis of the same side.

*ANALYSIS OF MOVEMENT*ius	*JOINTS*	*JOINT POSITION*	*MUSCLES STRETCHED*
Joint 1	Hip	Adduction, extension	Tensor fascia lata, sartor

EXERCISES

HIP AND BACK EXTENSION

Basic description:

- Inhale, draw your navel towards your spine, then slowly lift the chest, arms, head and legs from the floor as high as possible.
- Pause in the top position for up to three seconds.
- Then slowly return the arms and legs to the ground as you exhale.
- Repeat the process ten to twenty times.

Tips for good form:

- Keep your head in line with the spine (do not extend your head).
- Keep your arms out at 45° with the thumbs pointing upwards.

STARTING POSITION

- Lie face down with arms overhead at a 45° angle.
- Lengthen legs away from you and press tops of feet lightly into the floor, lifting the knees.
- Turn your thumbs up so you are resting on the outer edges of your hands.

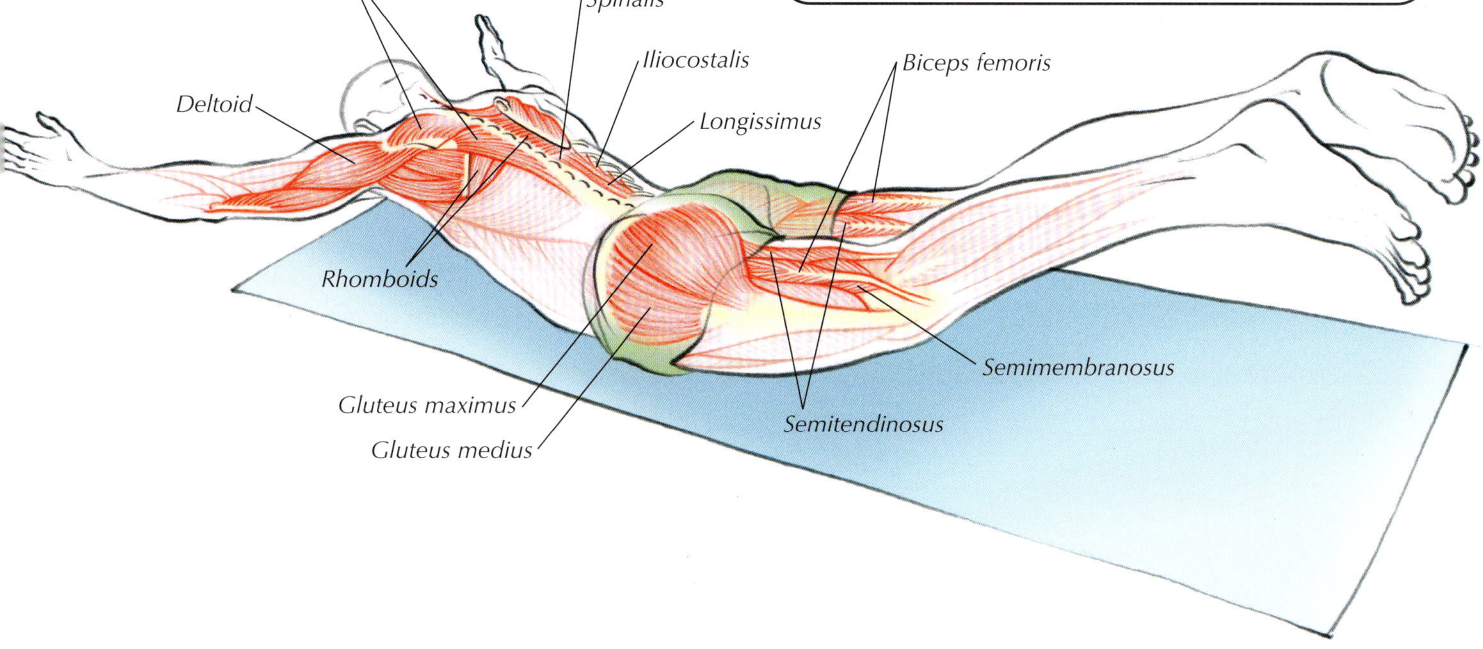

ANALYSIS OF MOVE-MENTres)	JOINTS	JOINT MOVEMENT	STABILIZING MUSCLES
Joint 1	Lumbar spine	Extension	Longissimus, iliocostalis, spinalis, quadratus lumborum, multifidus
Joint 2	Hip	Extension	Gluteus maximus, gluteus medius (posterior fibres), biceps femoris, semitendinosus, semimembranosus, adductor magnus (posterior fib

PRONE COBRA

Basic description:

- Inhale drawing your navel in towards your spine, and slowly lift chest, shoulders, hands and head from the floor by extending the upper back.
- Externally rotate your shoulders so your thumbs are pointing towards the ceiling.
- Keep the back of the neck long and your gaze to the floor.
- Hold the position for three minutes per set, resting during the set as required.

Tips for good form:

- Keep your head in line with the spine (do not extend the head).
- Squeeze your shoulder blades together and keep the shoulders down (away from the ears).

STARTING POSITION

- Lie face down with arms by the side with palms to floor.
- Rest your forehead on the floor.

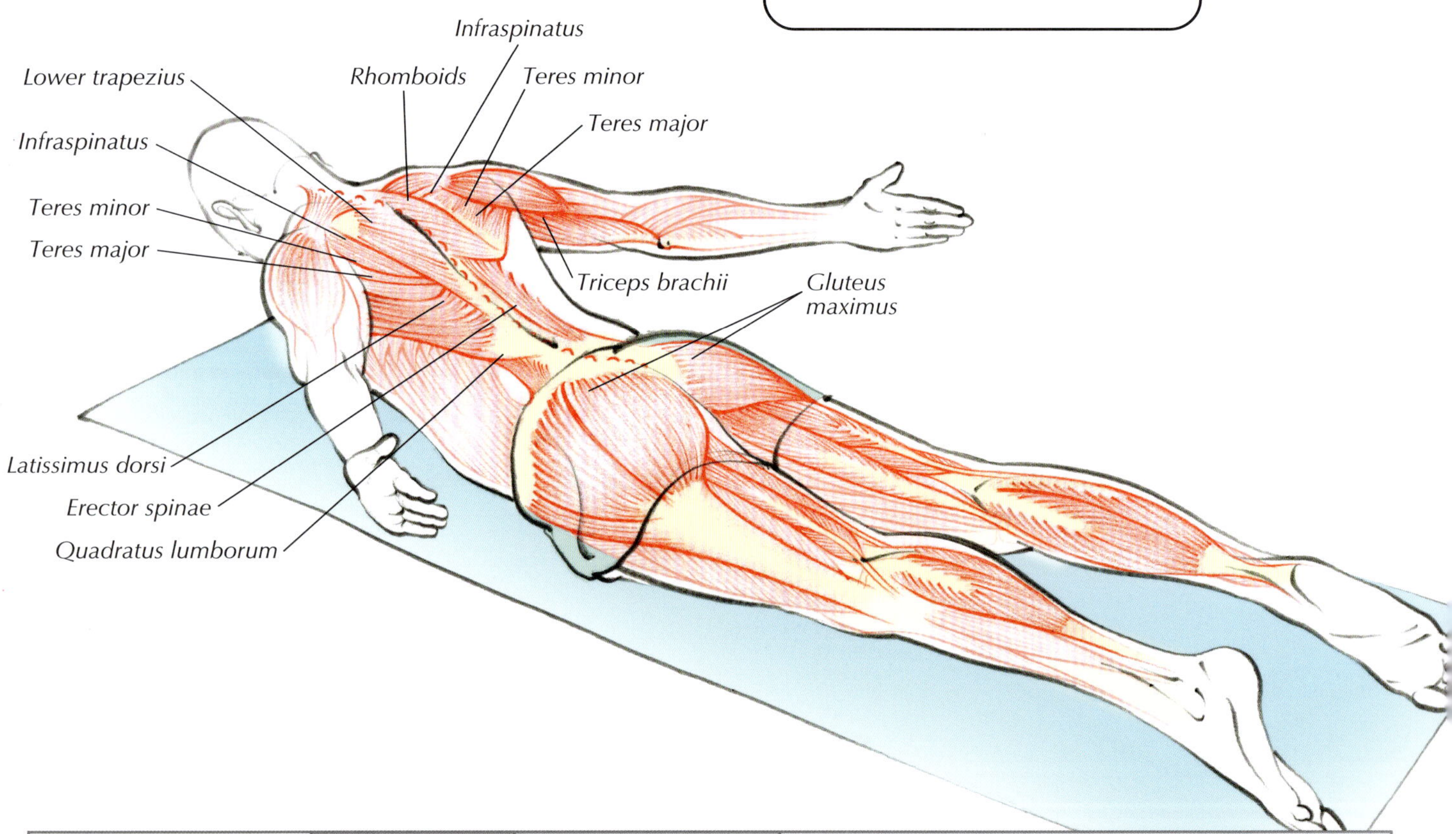

ANALYSIS OF MOVEMENT- natus	***JOINTS***	***JOINT MOVEMENT***	***STABILIZING MUSCLES***
Joint 1	Thoracic spine	Extension	Longissimus, iliocostalis, spinalis, semispinalis capitis, splenius cervicis, multifidus
Joint 2	Scapula	Adduction, depression	Rhomboids, trapezius (middle and inferior fibres), pectoralis minor
Joint 3	Shoulder	External rotation	Deltoid (posterior fibres), teres minor, infraspi

FOUR-POINT TUMMY VACUUM

Basic description:

- Inhale, allowing your abdomen to drop down towards the ground.
- As you exhale, gently draw the navel towards the spine, or imagine using the toilet and having to stop the flow (this activates your pelvic floor muscles), without any movement in the spine.
- Hold the contraction for 10 seconds.
- Inhale again and repeat for ten repetitions.

STARTING POSITION

- Position yourself on all fours (horse stance position).
- Your hands should be directly under the shoulders, with knees directly under the hips.
- A stick or dowel can be placed on the spine to help create a 'neutral spine'. The gap between the stick and the lumbar spine should be equal to the width of your hand.

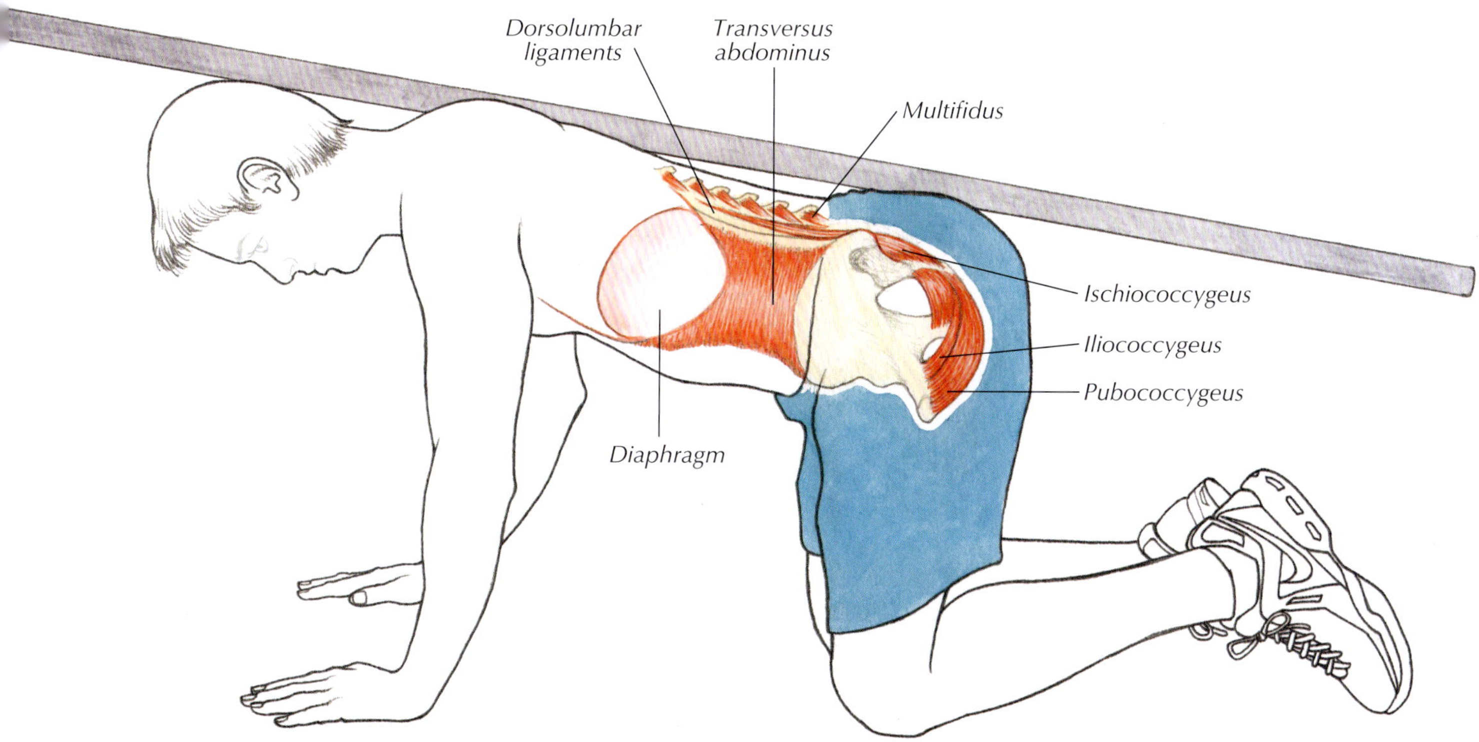

Tips for good form:

- Keep the spine in a neutral position.
- Ensure that as you breathe in, the abdomen drops towards the ground.

*ANALYSIS OF MOVEMENT*y-geus	*JOINTS*	*JOINT MOVEMENT*	*STABILIZING MUSCLES*
Joint 1	Rib cage	Stabilization	Diaphragm, transversus abdominus
Joint 2	Lumbar spine	Stabilization	Transversus abdominus, multifidus
Joint 3	Pelvis	Stabilization	Transversus abdominus, puborectalis, pubococcygeus, iliococcygeus, ischiococc

CABLE ROTATOR CUFF

Basic description (internal rotators):

- Start by standing side on to a cable machine. Grab the cable handle with the closest hand with your elbow tucked into your side.
- Inhale and gently draw your navel towards the spine.
- As you exhale, slowly draw the cable across your body as far as possible.
- From the finish position, return back to the start keeping the navel drawn in towards the spine. Inhale as you return back to the starting position.

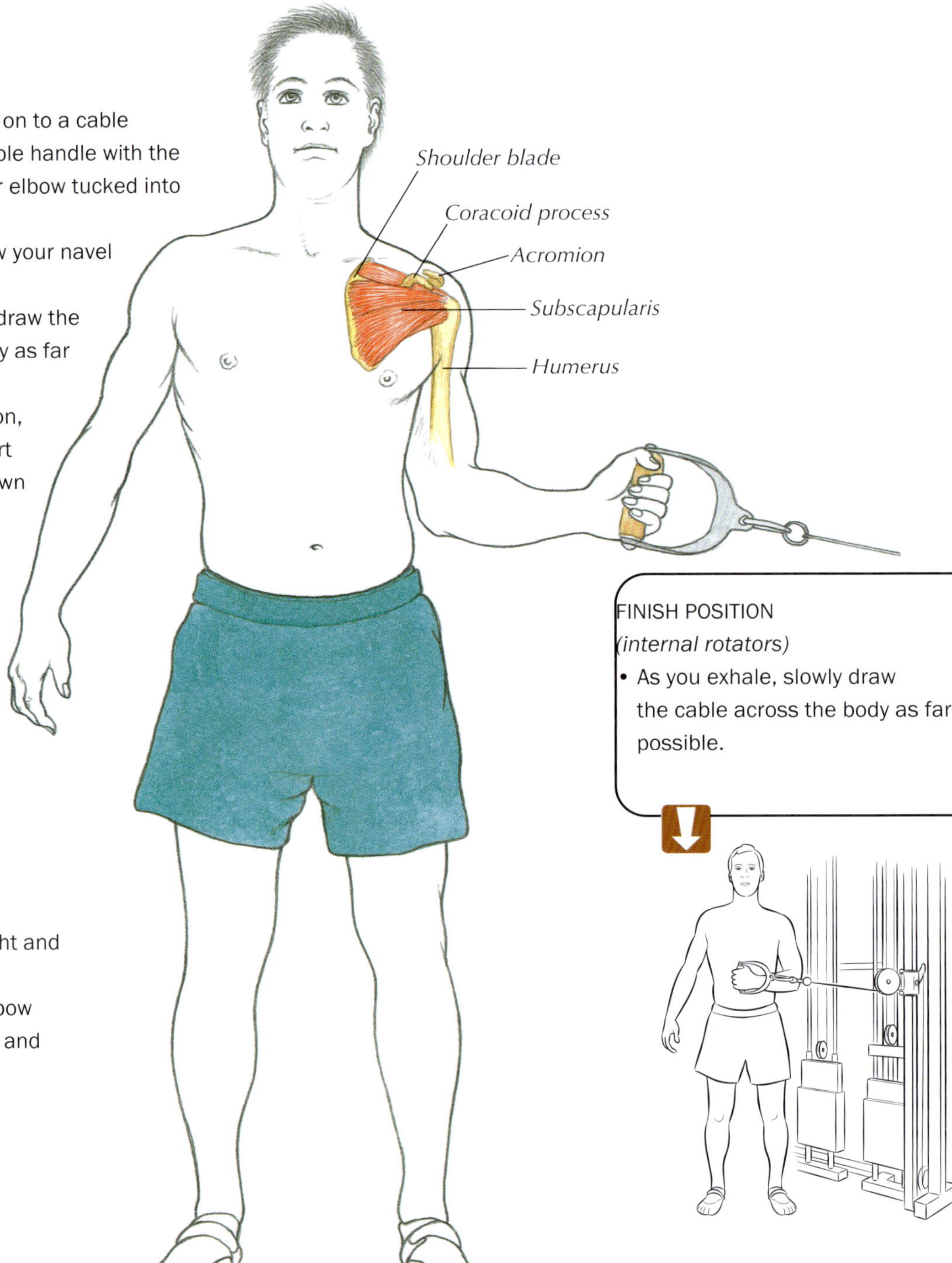

FINISH POSITION
(internal rotators)

- As you exhale, slowly draw the cable across the body as far as possible.

Tips for good form:

- Keep your torso upright and look straight ahead.
- Keep your working elbow tucked in to your side and bent to 90°.

ANALYSIS OF MOVEMEN-Trior	*JOINTS*	*JOINT MOVEMENT*	*MOBILIZING MUSCLES*
Joint 1	Shoulder	Internal rotation	Deltoid (anterior fibres), subscapularis, pectoralis major, latissimus dorsi, teres major.
Joint 2	Shoulder girdle (Scapula)	Adduction	Pectoralis minor, serratus ante

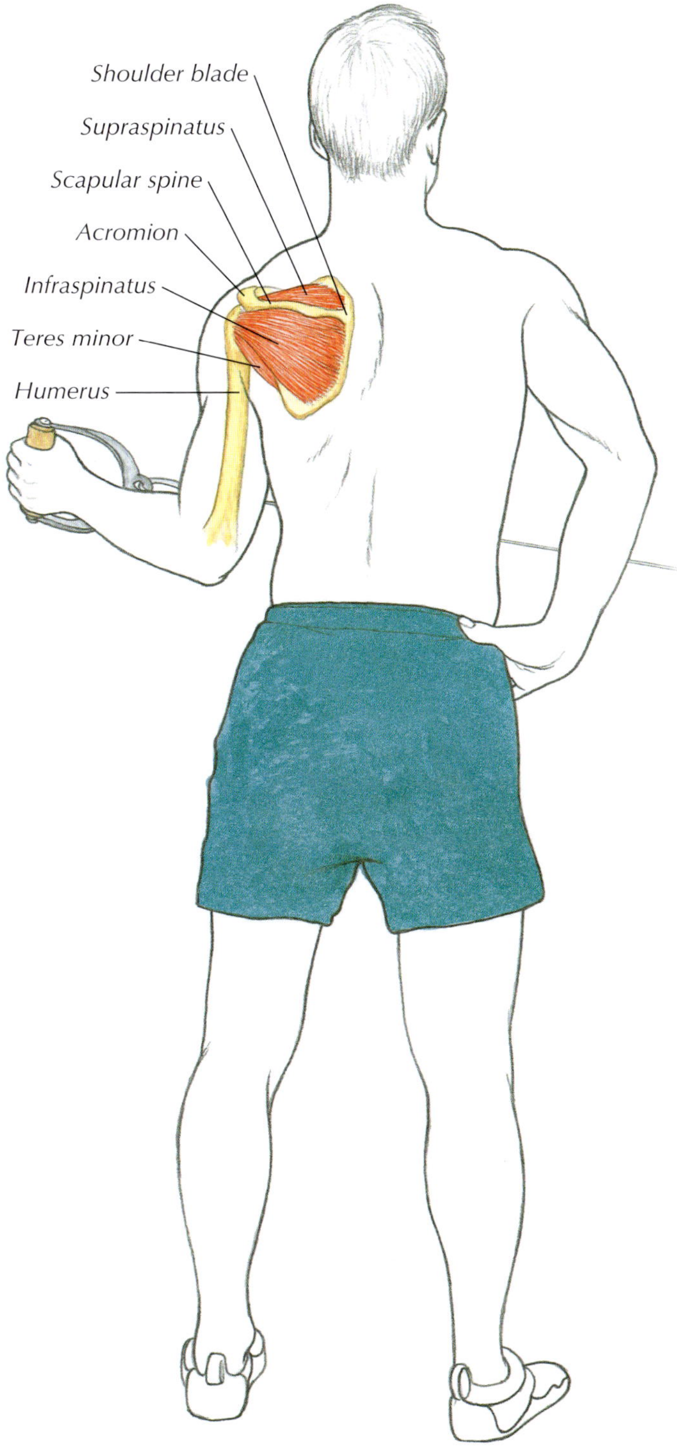

Basic description (external rotators):

- Gently draw your navel towards the spine.
- As you inhale, slowly draw the cable across the body as far as it will go.
- From the end position, return back to the start keeping the navel drawn in towards the spine. Exhale as you return back to the start position.

STARTING POSITION
(external rotators)

- Stand side on to a cable machine. Grab the cable handle with the furthest hand with the elbow tucked into the side.

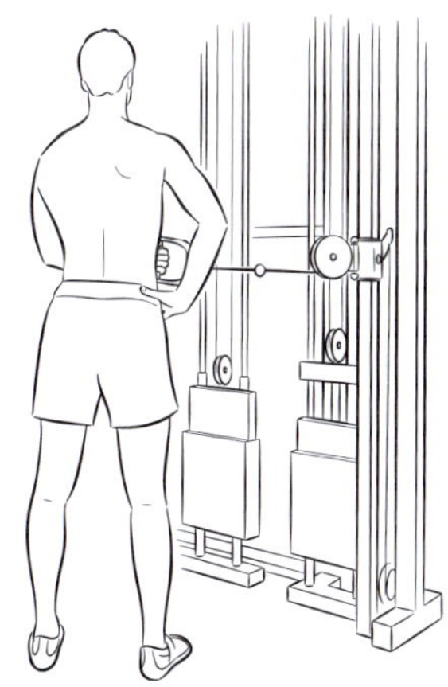

ANALYSIS OF MOVEMENT- bres	*JOINTS*	*JOINT MOVEMENT*	*MOBILIZING MUSCLES*
Joint 1	Shoulder	External rotation	Deltoid (posterior fibres), infraspinatus, teres minor
Joint 2	Shoulder girdle (Scapula)	Abduction	Rhomboids, Trapezius (middle fi

CROSS BAND WALKING

Basic description:

- Holding the crossed bands, begin walking forwards slowly.
- Each stride should exaggerate hip abduction, i.e. wide strides at a 45°-angle.

Tips for good form:

- Keep the torso upright, do not allow the torso to move side to side and continue looking straight ahead.
- Keep the palms facing forwards.

STARTING POSITION

- Place an exercise band under both feet.
- Hold each end of the band in your hands.
- Switch the ends into opposite hands, so they cross over.
- Stand upright with good posture, palms facing forwards.

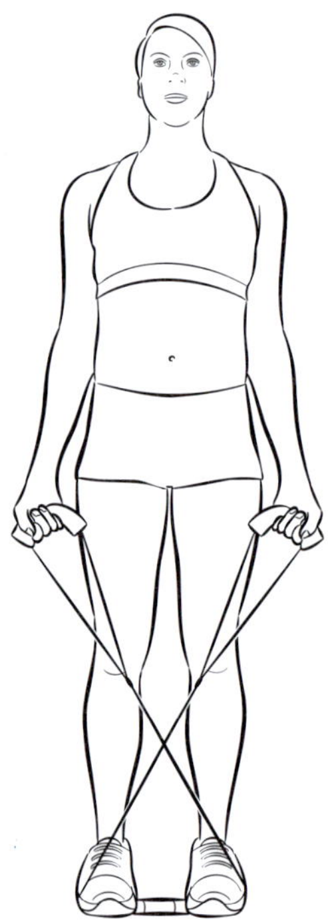

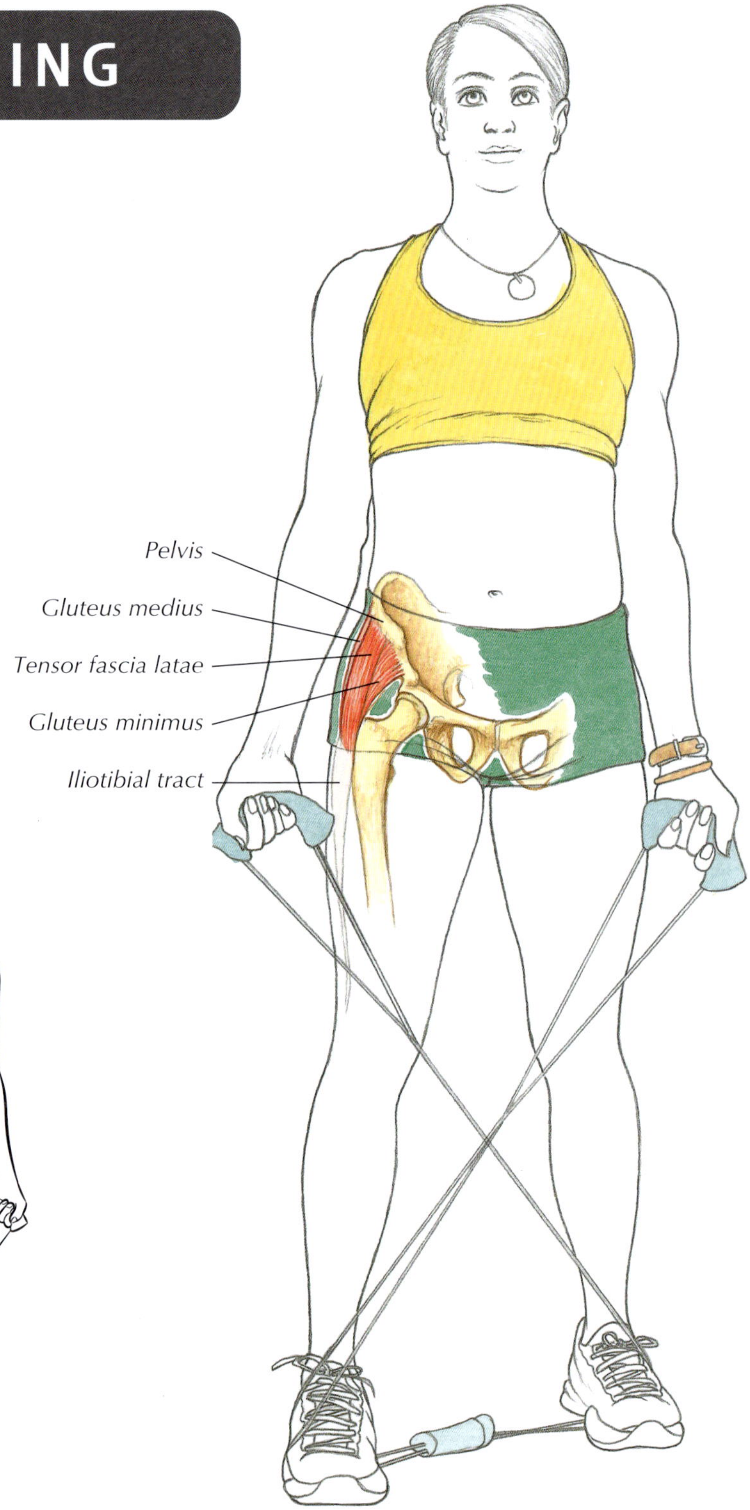

*ANALYSIS OF MOVEMENT*lis	*JOINTS*	*JOINT MOVEMENT*	*MOBILIZING MUSCLES*
Joint 1	Hip	Flexion, abduction	Gluteus medius (anterior and medial fibres), gluteus minimus, gluteus maximus, tensor facia lata, iliopsoas, rectus femoris, vastus medialis, vastus intermedius, vastus latera

DEEP CERVICAL FLEXORS

Basic description:

- Place your tongue on the roof of your mouth behind your front teeth.
- Tuck your chin in until the dial on the cuff increases by 10mmHg.
- Hold for 10 seconds or more, up to three minutes depending on your sport requirements for neck stability. Complete sets of total time under tension of 120 to 180 seconds.
- Contraindicated for people with a cervical disc bulge.

STARTING POSITION

- Lying on your back with your legs bent to 90°, place a blood pressure cuff or biofeedback unit under your neck
- Pump the cuff up to 30mmHg.

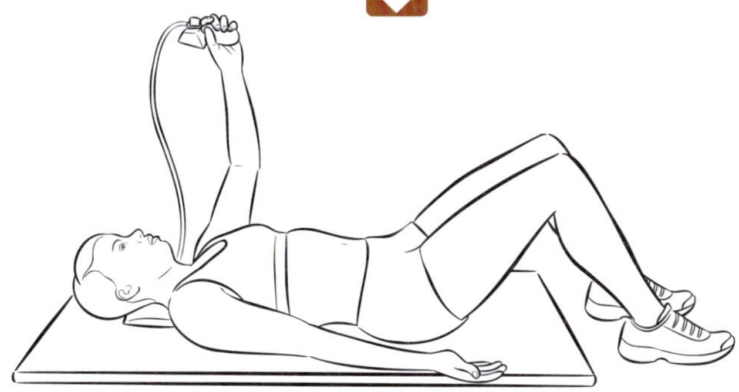

Tips for good form:

- Tuck your chin in, using an axis that runs through the middle of the ears (auditory meatus). Do not nod your head forwards.
- Keep your head straight. You may need someone to watch you do it for feedback.

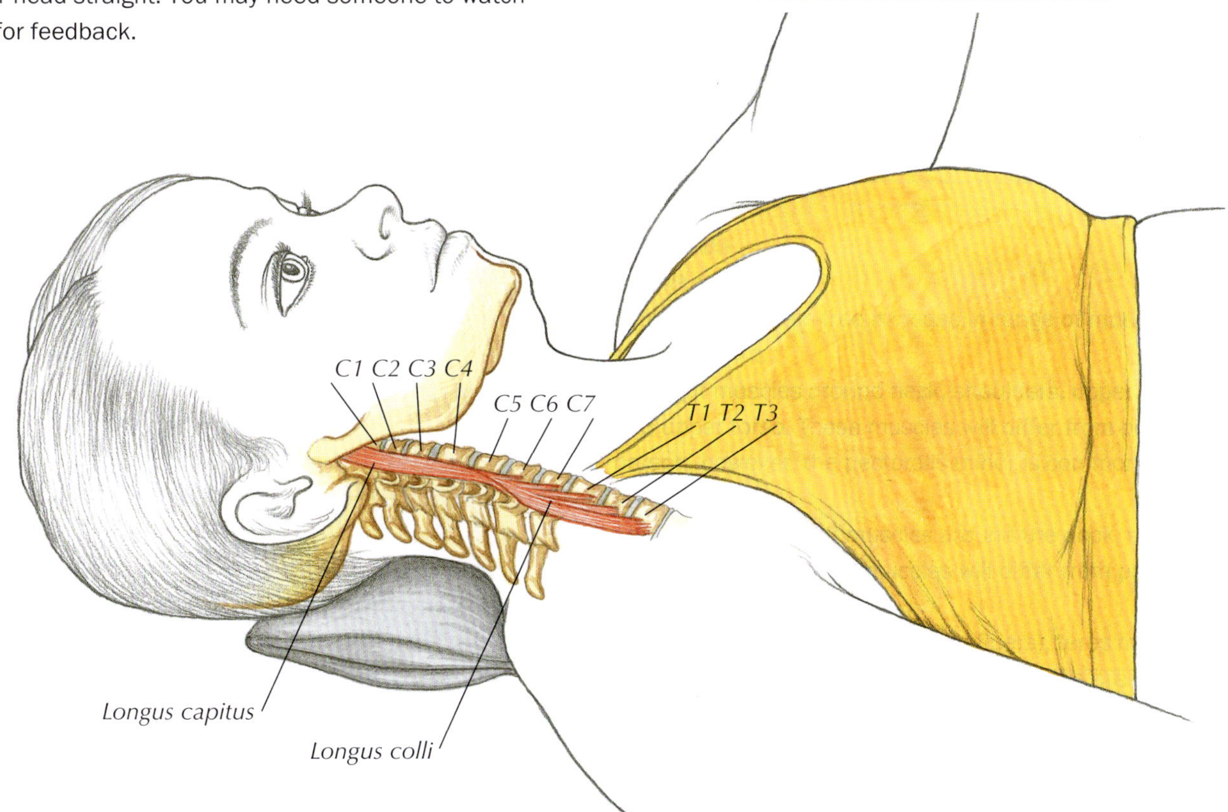

*ANALYSIS OF MOVEMENT*olli	*JOINTS*	*JOINT MOVEMENT*	*MOBILIZING MUSCLES*
Joint 1	Occipito-Atlanto	Cranial flexion	Longus capitis
Joint 2	Cervical Spine	Flexion	Longus capitiis, longus c

GOOF BALL NECK EXERCISES

Basic description:

- Place your tongue on the roof of the mouth behind the front teeth.
- Gently side-bend your head and neck into the ball using an intensity that you can hold easily for at least 30 seconds.
- Gently rotate your head and neck in the same way and hold.
- Gently extend your head and neck into the ball (by pushing away from a door frame) and hold.
- Gently flex your head and neck into the ball (by pulling towards you on the post/door frame) and hold.
- Repeat each position two to six times per set.

Tips for good form:

- Keep your whole body in good postural alignment.
- Use a gentle intensity.
- Use your eyes to aid the movement of the muscles, i.e. eyes down with flexion, eyes to side that you are side-flexing and rotating to, and eyes up when extending.

STARTING POSITIONS

- Standing up straight with a Goof Ball placed on the side of the head (side flexion or rotation), at the back of the head (extension), or on the forehead (flexion).
- The Goof Ball should be supported against a wall or fixed post or doorframe. Hold on to the doorframe or post for support.

Side flexion or rotation **Flexion** **Extension**

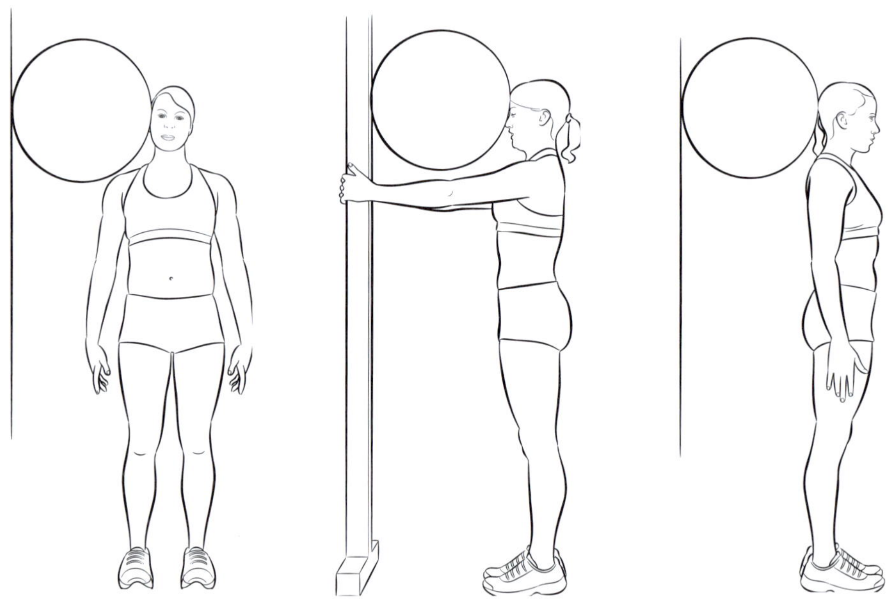

*ANALYSIS OF MOVEMENT*ibres)	*JOINTS*	*JOINT MOVEMENT*	*MOBILIZING MUSCLES*
Joint 1Cervical		Side flexion	Splenius capitis, splenius cervicis, longus capitis, longus colli
		Rotation	Ipsilateral: rectus capitis posterior major, oblique capitis inferior, longus capitis, longus colli, levator scapula, splenius capitis, splenius cervicis Contralateral: trapezius (upper fibres), sternocleidomastoid, scalenes
		Extension	Splenius capitis, splenius cervicis, Rectus capitis posterior major and minor, oblique capitis superior.
		Flexion	Longus capitis, longus colli, scalenes (anterior f

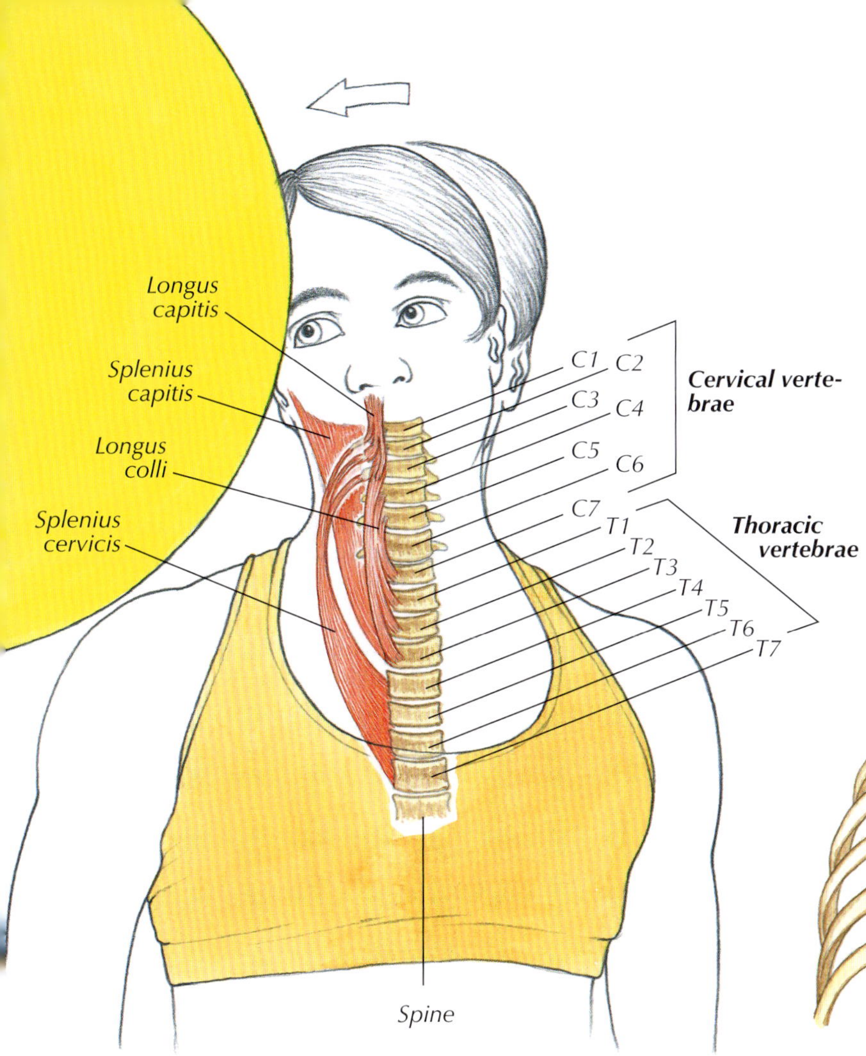

Side flexion

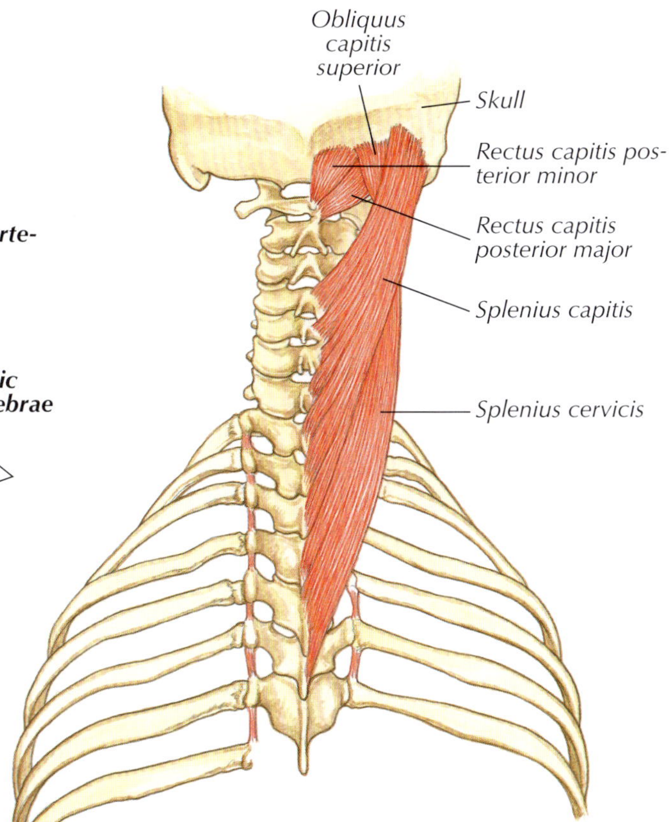

Extension

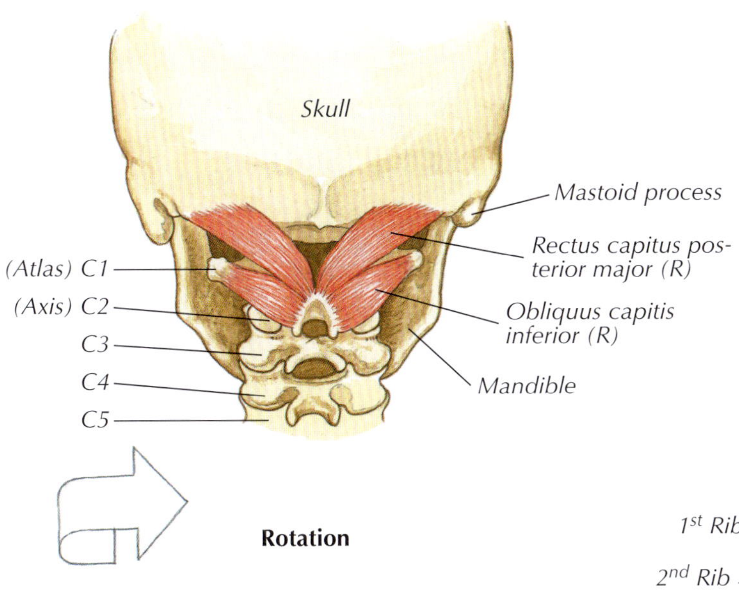

Rotation

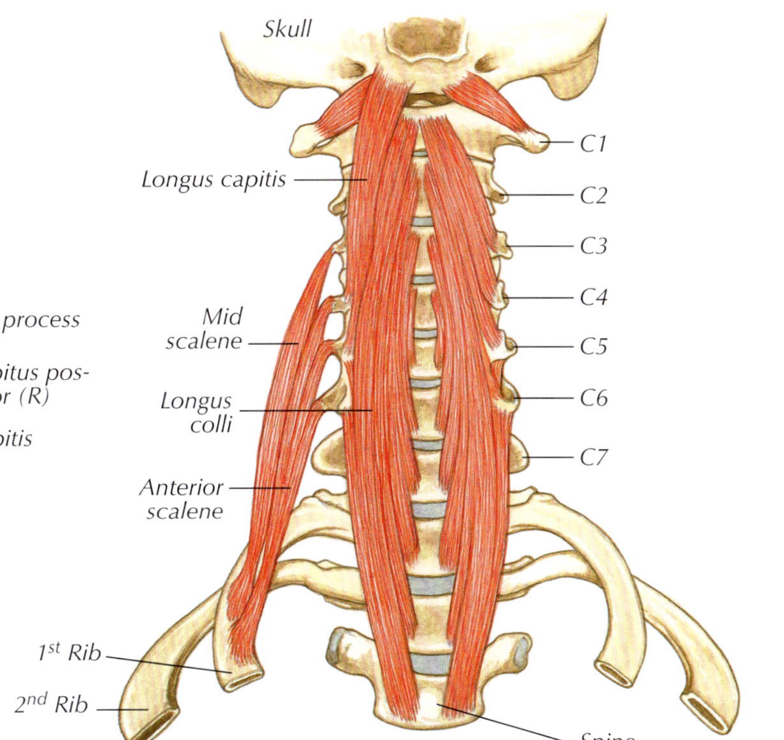

Flexion

HORSE STANCE VERTICAL

STARTING POSITION

- Position yourself on all fours (horse stance position).
- Your hands should be directly under your shoulders, with knees directly under your hips.
- A stick or dowel can be placed on the spine to help create a 'neutral' spine. The gap between the stick and the lumbar spine should be equal to the width of your hand.

Basic description:

- Inhale, allowing the abdomen to drop down towards the ground.
- As you exhale, gently draw your navel towards the spine or imagine using the toilet and having to stop the flow (this activates your pelvic floor muscles), without any movement in the spine.
- Simultaneously, raise one hand and the opposite knee a millimetre off the floor. Keep the spine in neutral and try to avoid any twisting of the spine or any side-to-side movement of the torso or hips.
- Hold the contraction for five to ten seconds. Then switch sides for five to ten seconds.
- Breathe naturally while continuing to draw in your navel and repeating ten times on each side.

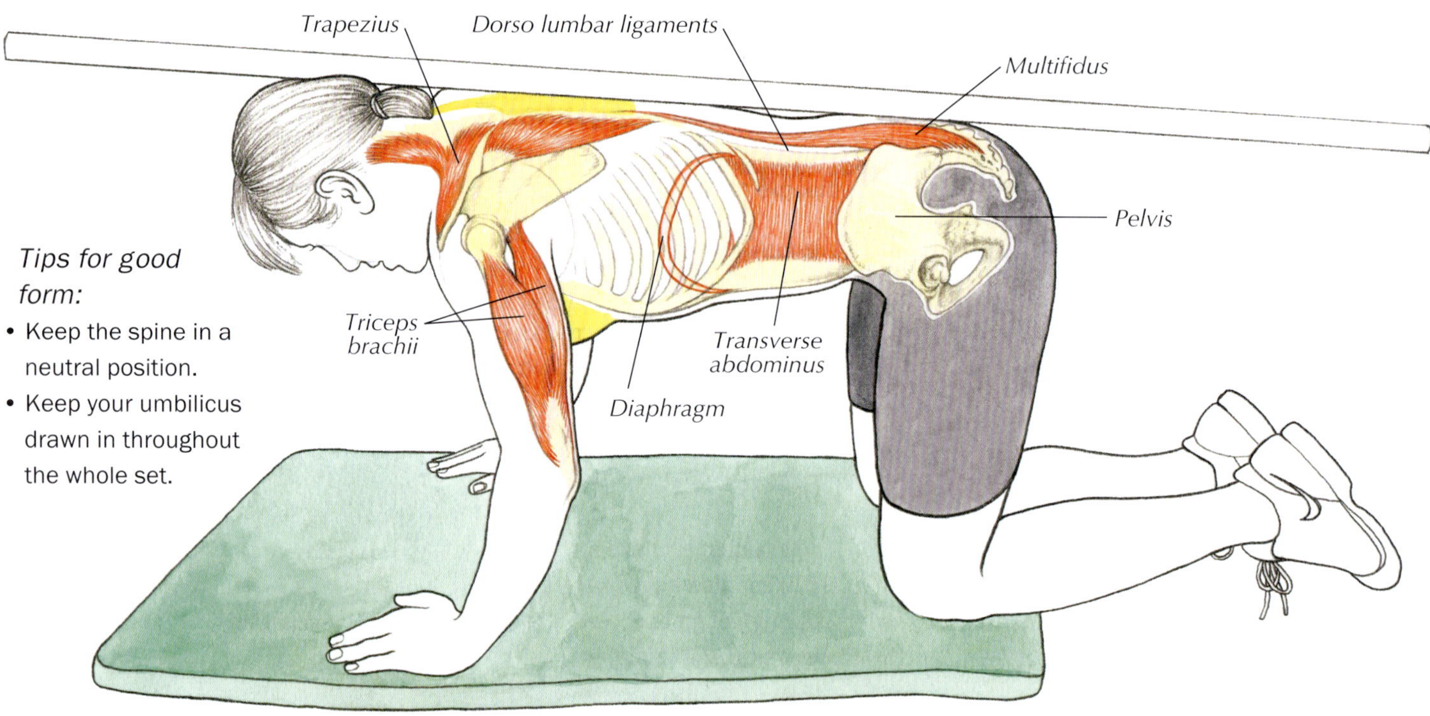

Tips for good form:

- Keep the spine in a neutral position.
- Keep your umbilicus drawn in throughout the whole set.

*ANALYSIS OF MOVEMENT*ed side)	*JOINTS*	*JOINT MOVEMENT*	*WORKING MUSCLES*
Joint 1	Rib cage	Stabilization	Diaphragm, transversus abdominus
Joint 2	Lumbar spine	Stabilization	Transversus abdominus, multifidus
		Rotation	External and internal obliques, rotatores
Joint 3	Pelvis	Stabilization	Transversus abdominus, puborectalis, pubococcygeus, iliococcygeus, ischiococcygeus
Joint 4	Scapula	Adduction	Trapezius (middle fibres), rhomboid major and minor (lifted side)
Joint 5	Elbow	Stabilization	Triceps brachii (ground

LOWER ABDOMINALS

Basic description:

- Inhale into the abdomen, then exhale. As you exhale, gently draw your navel in towards the spine.
- Keeping the navel drawn in, flatten your back into the cuff until you increase the pressure by 30mmHg.
- Holding the pressure on the cuff, raise one leg (start with knees bent) until the knee points to the ceiling. Alternate legs.
- You can progress the exercise by straightening the legs. You can start with both legs up and then lower them one at a time to do the exercise. You can raise both legs together.
- The aim is to strengthen the lower abdominals as quickly as possible. Floor exercise should only be continued until the muscles are strong enough to allow good form in standing exercises.

Tips for good form:

- Keep navel drawn in towards the spine.
- Keep the pressure on the dial in the exact position. Movement of the dial equals poor form.
- Check angles of your spinal curves, ideally before beginning this exercise and at four weeks to ensure you do not flatten your lumbar spine with this exercise.

STARTING POSITION

- Lying supine, legs bent to 90°, place a blood pressure cuff or biofeedback unit in the small of your lower back.
- Pump the cuff up to 40mmHg.

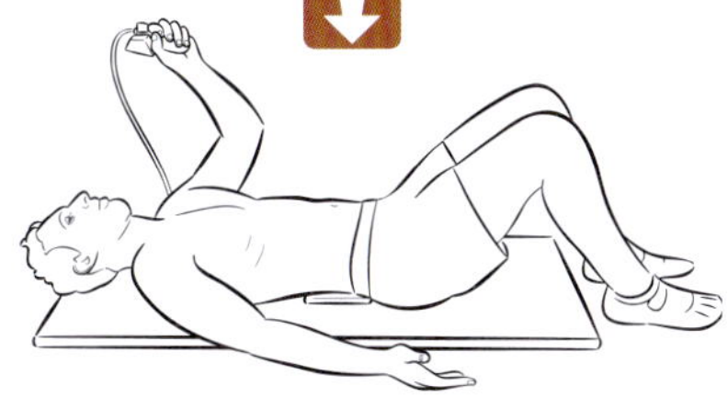

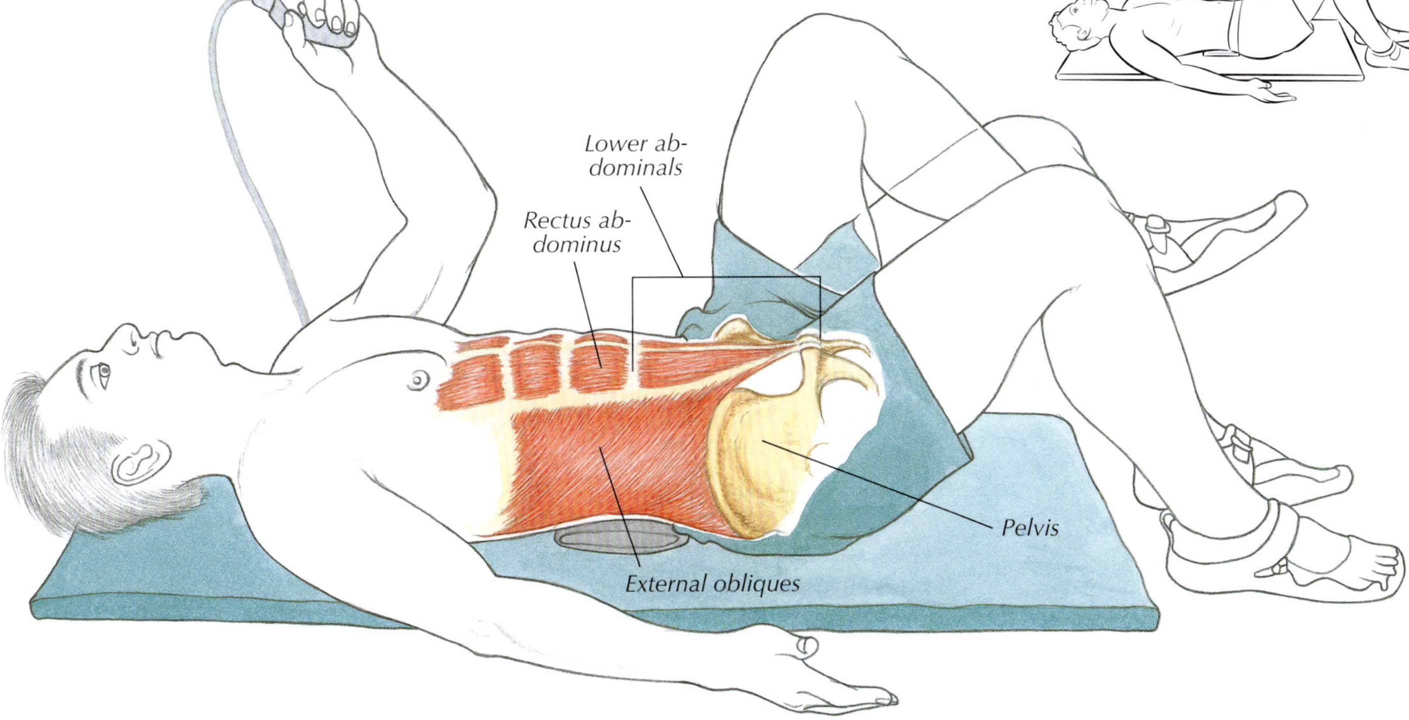

ANALYSIS OF MOVEMEN-Troup	*JOINTS*	*JOINT MOVEMENT*	*WORKING MUSCLES*
Joint 1	Hip	Hip flexion	Iliopsaos, rectus femoris, tensor fascia lata, adductors
Joint 2	Lumbo-pelvic	Flexion	External obliques, rectus abdominus, transversus abdominus, gluteus maximus, hamstrings g

STAND/SQUAT ON BALANCE BOARD

STARTING POSITION

- Stand on a balance board with your torso upright and eyes looking straight ahead.
- Feet shoulder-width apart and can be turned out up to 30°.

Basic description:

- Inhale, gently drawing your navel in towards the spine.
- Initially, just stand while maintaining good balance.
- When you feel confident enough, descend into a squat position, like sitting in a chair, as far as you can without rounding (flexing) your lumbar spine.
- At the bottom of the squat, slowly drive your heels through the balance board to drive you back up.
- Exhale through the most challenging part of the ascent.

Tips for good form:

- Keep the torso upright, look straight ahead.
- Keep the knees in line with the second toe on each foot.

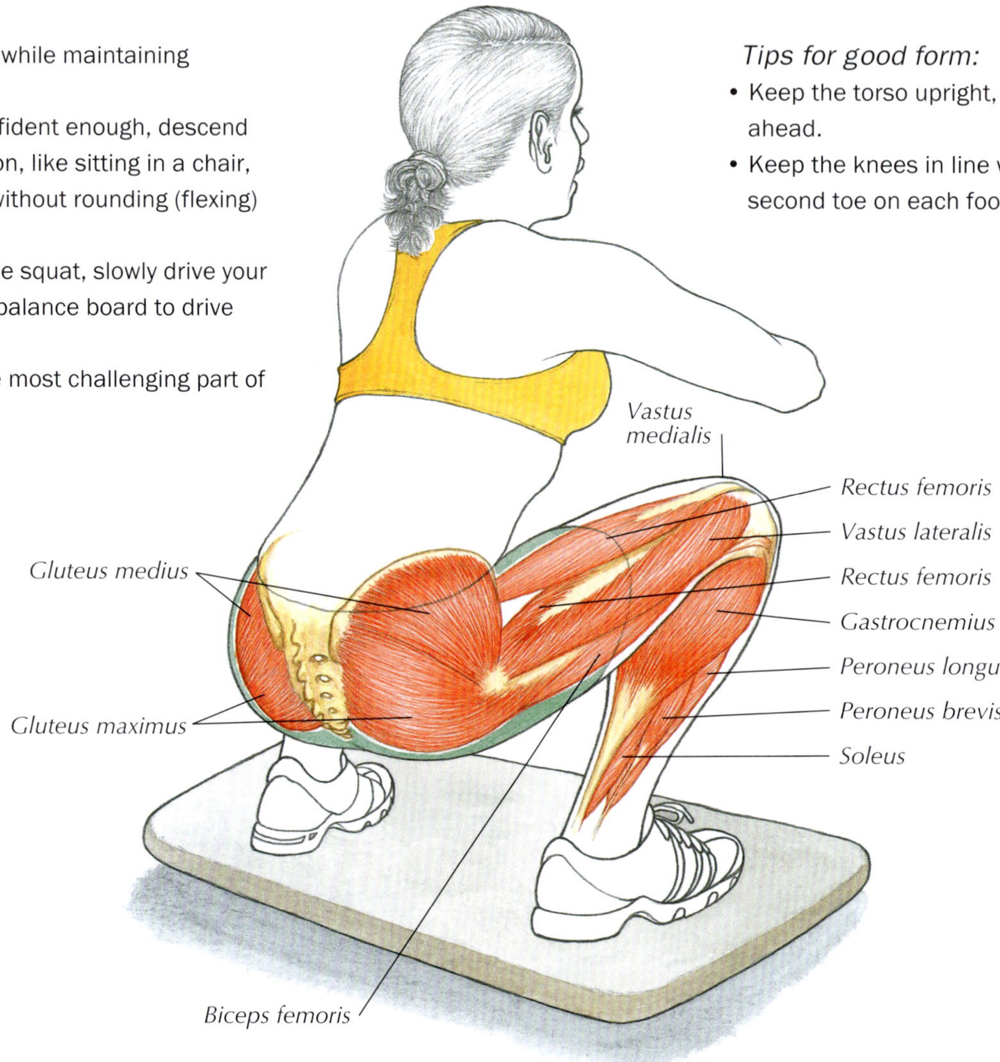

ANALYSIS OF MOVEMENTre-vis	JOINTS	JOINT MOVEMENT	MOBILIZING MUSCLES
Joint 1	Hip	Down: Flexion Up: Extension	Gluteus maximus, gluteus medius (posterior fibres), biceps femoris, semitendinosus, semimembranosus, adductor magnus (posterior fibres)
Joint 2	Knee	Down: Flexion Up: Extension	Rectus femoris, vastus medialis, vastus intermedius, vastus lateralis
Joint 3	Ankle	Down: Dorsiflexion Up: Plantarflexion	Gastrocnemius, soleus, tibialis posterior, peroneus longus and b

SUPINE LATERAL BALL ROLL

Basic description:

- Inhale, gently drawing your navel in towards the spine.
- Shuffle sideways on the ball to the point where you can just keep good posture and balance. Hold for one to three seconds. Repeat on the other side.

Tips for good form:

- Keep your head and torso straight (no side-bending) and shoulders and hips parallel to the ground and spine in neutral alignment.
- Keep your shins perpendicular to the floor and keep your hips at the same height as the shoulders, but avoid arching your lower back.
- Do not let your knees move forwards of the ankles.

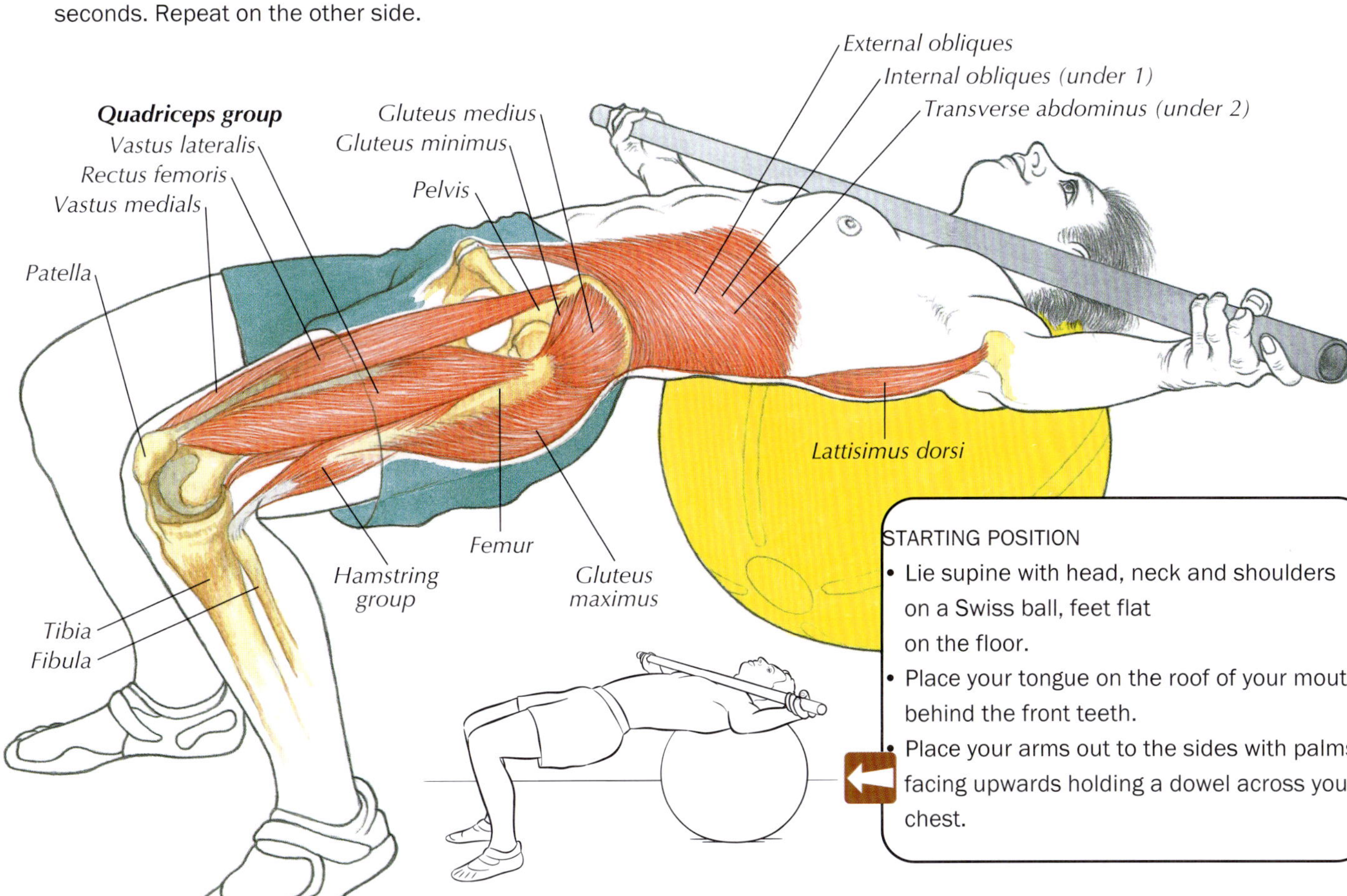

STARTING POSITION

- Lie supine with head, neck and shoulders on a Swiss ball, feet flat on the floor.
- Place your tongue on the roof of your mouth behind the front teeth.
- Place your arms out to the sides with palms facing upwards holding a dowel across your chest.

*ANALYSIS OF MOVEMENT*aris	*JOINTS*	*JOINT MOVEMENT*	*MOBILIZING AND MAJOR STABILIZING MUSCLES*
Joint 1	Spine	Stabilization	Transversus abdominus, multifidus, rotatores, internal obliques, external obliques, Longus capitis, longus colli, scalenes, splenius capitis, splenius cervicis, longus capitis, longus colli, rectus capitis posterior major, oblique capitis inferior, longus capitis, longus colli
Joint 2	Hip	Stabilization	Gluteus maximus, gluteus medius, gluteus minimus, tensor fascia lata, gracilis, pectineus, adductor longus, adductor brevis, adductor magnus
Joint 3	Knee	Stabilization	Rectus femoris, vastus medialis, vastus intermedius, vastus lateralis, biceps femoris, semitendinosus, semimembranosus, gastrocnemius, gracilis, sartorius, popliteus, plant

TOUCH TOE DRILL

Basic description:

- Inhale, then gently draw your navel in towards your spine.
- Keeping your standing foot fully on the ground, bend the same knee, then reach with the other foot as far forwards as possible.
- Tap the moving foot on the floor at the furthest point you can reach without placing any body weight on the moving foot.
- Repeat at 45° forwards, sideways, 45° backwards, and straight back.
- Repeat on the other side.

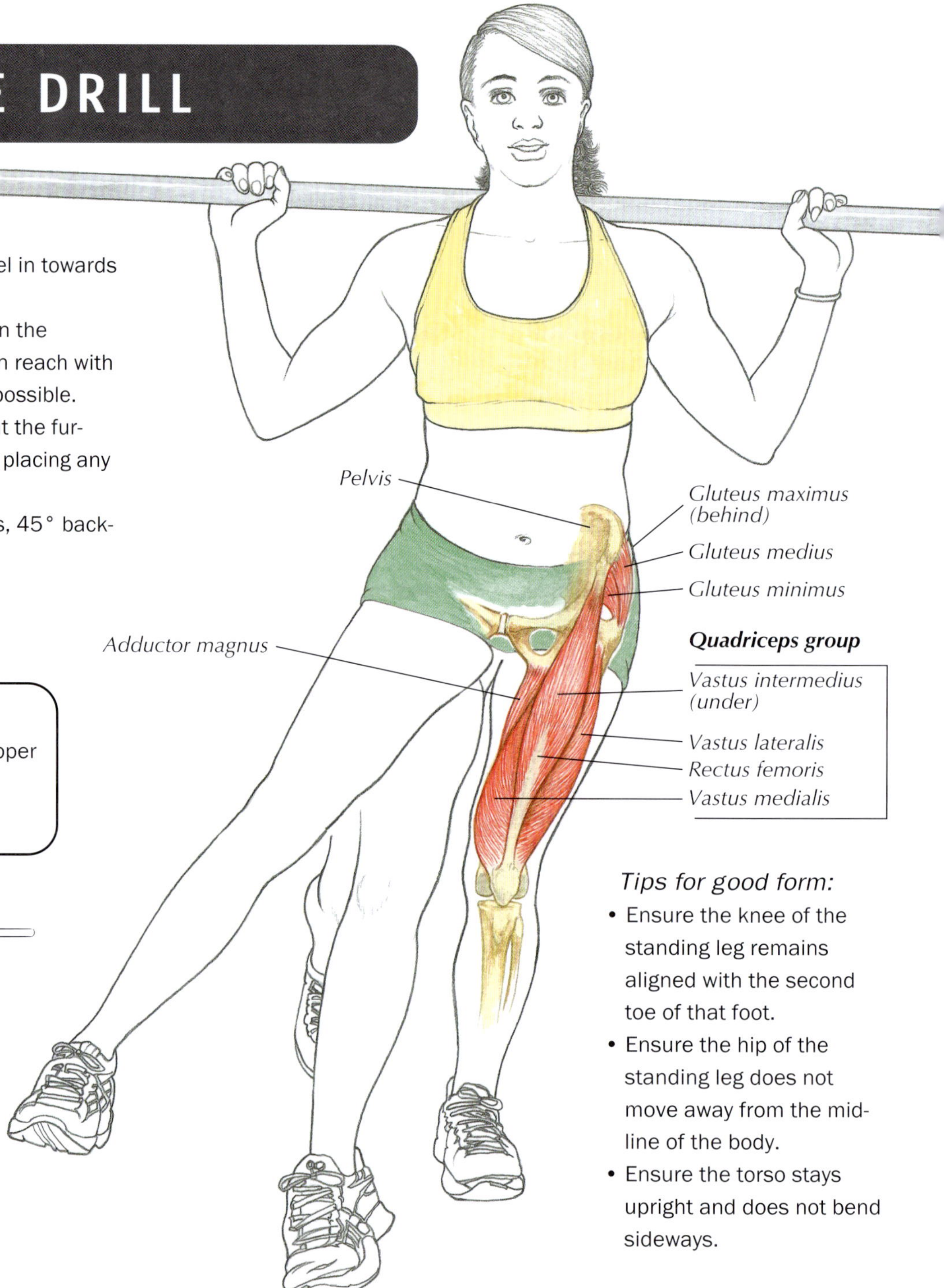

STARTING POSITION

- Stand with a dowel across your upper back, then lift one leg.

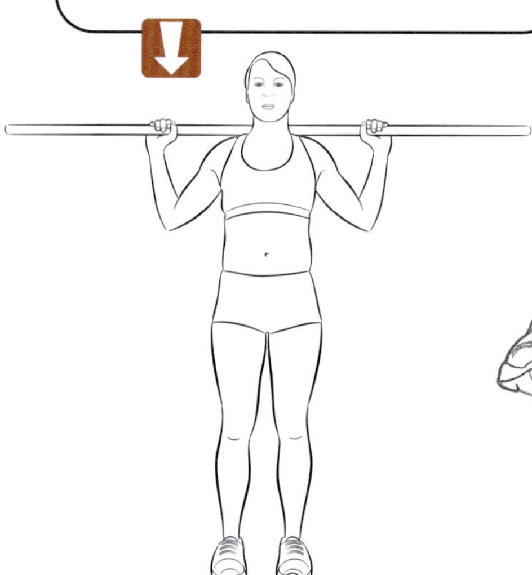

Tips for good form:

- Ensure the knee of the standing leg remains aligned with the second toe of that foot.
- Ensure the hip of the standing leg does not move away from the midline of the body.
- Ensure the torso stays upright and does not bend sideways.

*ANALYSIS OF MOVEMENT*re-vis	*JOINTS*	*JOINT MOVEMENT*	*MOBILIZING MUSCLES*
Joint 1	Hip	Up: extension Down: flexion	Gluteus maximus, gluteus medius (posterior fibres), biceps femoris, semitendinosus, semimembranosus, adductor magnus (posterior fibres)
Joint 2	Knee	Up: extension Down: flexion	Rectus femoris, vastus medialis, vastus intermedius, vastus lateralis
Joint 3	Ankle	Up: plantarflexion Down: dorsiflexion	Gastrocnemius, soleus, tibialis posterior, peroneus longus and b

DEADLIFT

Basic description:

- Inhale, then draw your navel towards the spine.
- Drive your feet through the floor to initiate the ascent, exhaling through pursed lips through the most challenging part of the lift. Keep the torso at the same angle until the bar passes your knees.
- Keep the bar as close to your body as possible as you lift.
- As soon as the weight passes the knees, drive the hips forwards until you are standing upright. Keep your arms straight throughout.
- At the top of the exercise, keep the navel drawn in and inhale. Then descend the weight, keeping it close to the body by bending at the hips until the weight reaches the knees, then bend the knees until the weight reaches the floor.
- Exhale through the most challenging part of the ascent and the descent.

Tips for good form:

- Ensure the lumbar spine does not flex. You can tape your lumbar spine with athletic tape, so that you know if your spine is flexing.
- Keep a neutral spine and gently draw the shoulder blades together.
- Keep your eyes level with the horizon.

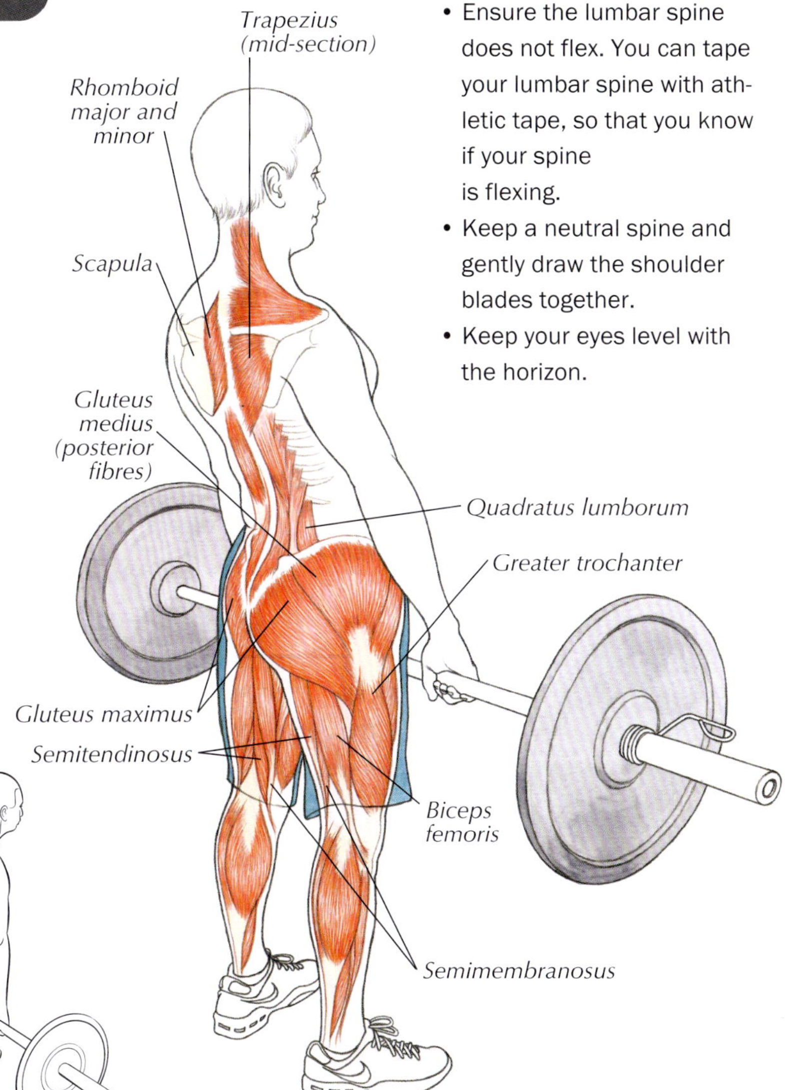

STARTING POSITION

- Use a bent forward position with a barbell in front of you, feet shoulder-width apart.
- Grip the bar and keep your spine in good alignment

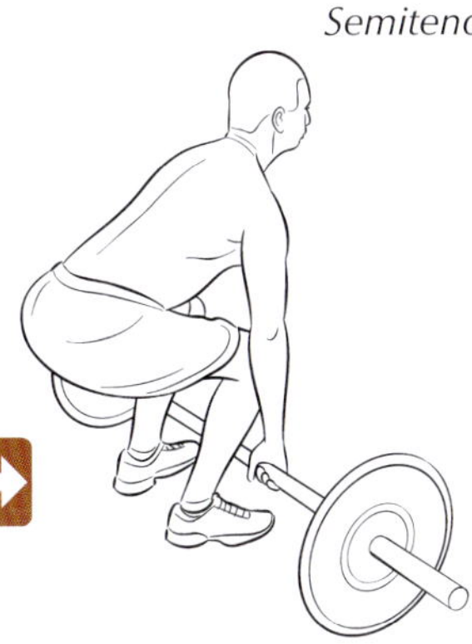

ANALYSIS OF MOVEMENT- ficialis	*JOINTS*	*JOINT MOVEMENT*	*MOBILIZING MUSCLES*
Joint 1	Hip	Up: extension Down: flexion	Gluteus maximus, gluteus medius (posterior fibres), biceps femoris, semitendinosus, semimembranosus, adductor magnus (posterior fibres)
Joint 2	Knee	Up: extension Down: flexion	Rectus femoris, vastus medialis, vastus intermedius, vastus lateralis
Joint 3	Ankle	Up: plantarflexion Down dorsiflexion	Gastrocnemius, soleus, tibialis posterior, peroneus longus and brevis
Joint 4	Lumbar Spine	Stabilization: extension	Multifidus, spinalis, longissimus, iliocostalis, quadratus lumborum, interspinalis
Joint 5	Scapula	Adduction	Trapezius (middle fibres), rhomboid major and minor
Joint 6	Wrist	Grip: flexion	Flexor carpi radialis, flexor carpi ulnaris, palmaris longus, flexor digitorum super

LUNGE (SPLIT SQUAT)

Basic description:

- Inhale, gently drawing the navel towards the spine.
- Take a large step forwards and lower the body down to the ground under control.
- Allow the knees to bend and finish with the back knee about an inch from the floor.
- Keep most of the weight on the front leg.
- At the bottom of the lunge, drive straight back up to the starting position by driving the front heel through the floor, exhaling through pursed lips as you pass through the most difficult part of the ascent.

Tips for good form:

- Keep the torso upright, gently squeeze your shoulder blades together and keep your head level with the horizon.
- Keep the front knee in line with the second toe as you descend and ascend. Do not allow the foot, ankle or knee to move towards the midline.
- Keep your weight on the mid to rear portion of your front foot.

STARTING POSITION

- Begin with a dumbbell in each hand, your torso upright and feet shoulder-width apart.
- Take a long stride forwards with one leg.

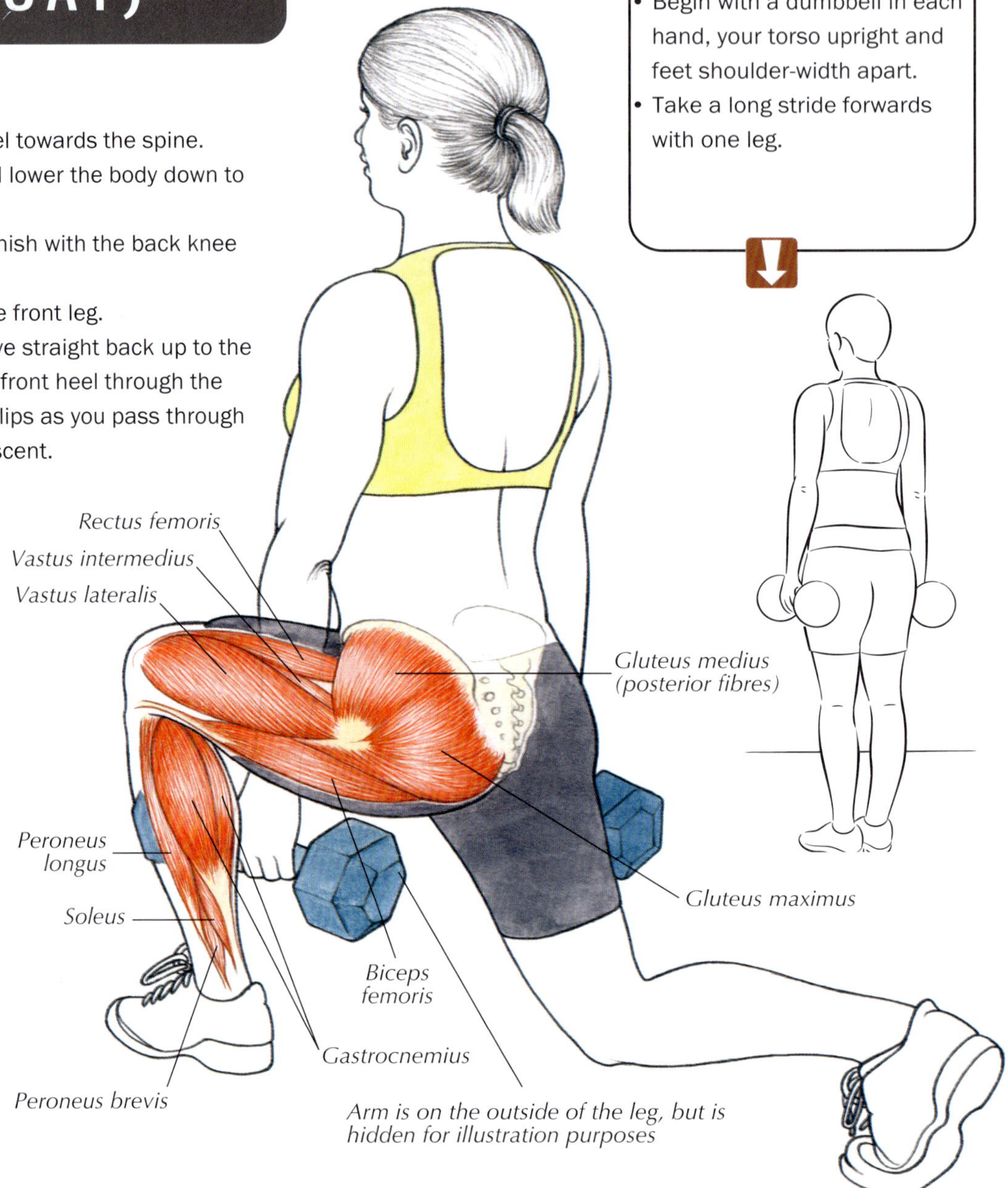

*ANALYSIS OF MOVEMENT*re-vis	*JOINTS*	*JOINT MOVEMENT*	*MOBILIZING MUSCLES*
Joint 1	Hip	Down: flexion Up: extension	Front leg: gluteus maximus, gluteus medius (posterior fibres), biceps femoris, semitendinosus, semimembranosus, adductor magnus (posterior fibres)
Joint 2	Knee	Down: flexion Up: extension	Front leg: rectus femoris, vastus medialis, vastus intermedius, vastus lateralis
Joint 3	Ankle	Down: dorsiflexion Up: plantarflexion	Front leg: gastrocnemius, soleus, tibialis posterior, peroneus longus and b

MEDICINE BALL SHOULDER EXTERNAL ROTATORS

Basic description:

- Throw the medicine ball backwards at the middle of the rebounder by rotating the shoulder and flicking your wrist.
- As your rehabilitation progresses and the tissues strengthen, you can also catch the medicine ball on the way back and immediately re-throw.

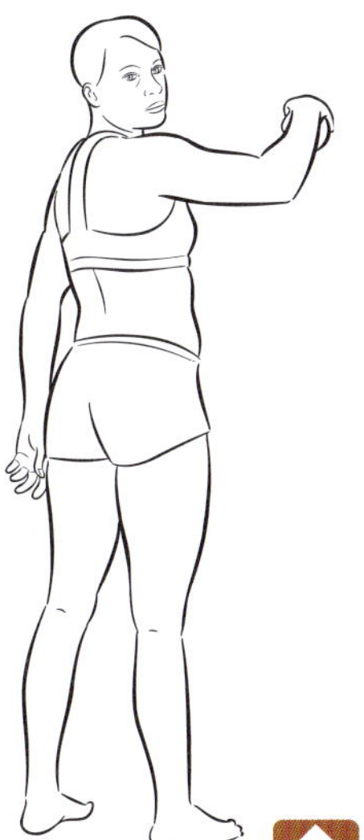

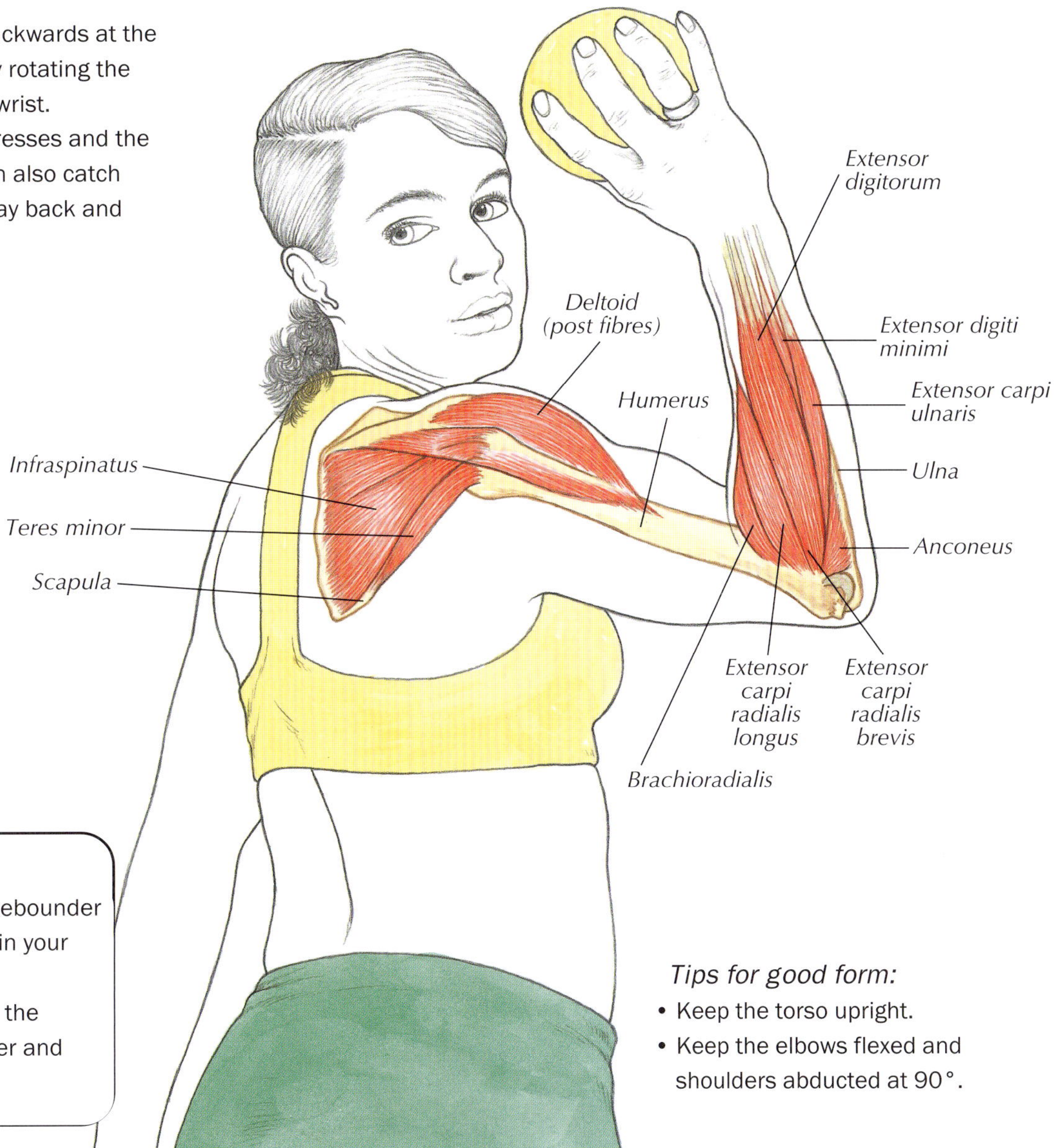

STARTING POSITION

- Stand facing away from a rebounder with a small medicine ball in your hand.
- Look over your shoulder at the rebounder with the shoulder and elbows flexed at 90°.

Tips for good form:

- Keep the torso upright.
- Keep the elbows flexed and shoulders abducted at 90°.

ANALYSIS OF MOVEMENT- naris	*JOINTS*	*JOINT MOVEMENT*	*MOBILIZING MUSCLES*
Joint 1	Shoulder	External rotation	Deltoid (posterior fibres), infraspinatus, teres minor
Joint 2	Shoulder girdle (Scapula)	Adduction	Rhomboids, trapezius (middle fibres)
Joint 3	Wrist	Extension	Extensor carpi radialis longus and brevis, extensor carpi ul

MEDICINE BALL SHOULDER INTERNAL ROTATORS

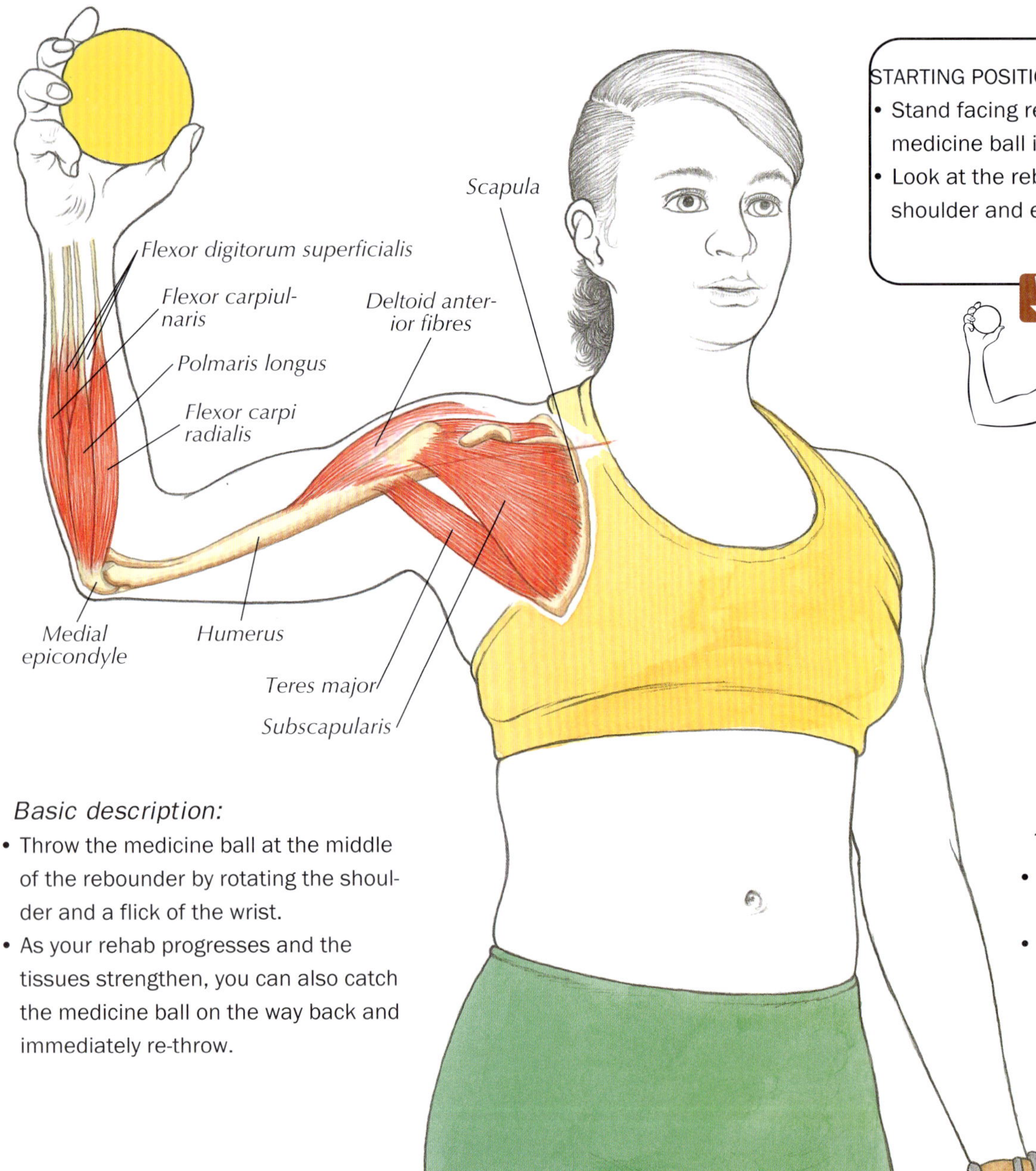

STARTING POSITION
- Stand facing rebounder with small medicine ball in hand.
- Look at the rebounder, with your shoulder and elbows flexed at 90°.

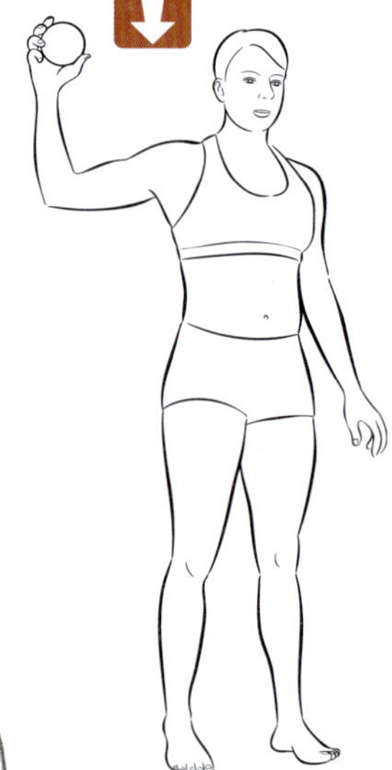

Basic description:
- Throw the medicine ball at the middle of the rebounder by rotating the shoulder and a flick of the wrist.
- As your rehab progresses and the tissues strengthen, you can also catch the medicine ball on the way back and immediately re-throw.

Tips for good form:
- Keep your torso and head upright.
- Keep the elbows flexed and shoulders abducted at 90°.

ANALYSIS OF MOVEMEN-Tialis	*JOINTS*	*JOINT MOVEMENT*	*MOBILIZING MUSCLES*
Joint 1	Shoulder	Internal rotation	Deltoid (anterior fibres), subscapularis
Joint 2	Shoulder girdle (Scapula)	Abduction	Pectoralis minor, serratus anterior
Joint 3	Wrist	Flexion	Flexor carpi radialis, flexor carpi ulnaris, palmaris longus, flexor digitorum superfic

ROMANIAN DEADLIFT (STIFF-LEG DEADLIFT)

Basic description:

- Inhale, drawing the navel towards the spine.
- With a slight bend in the knee and keeping a 'neutral spine', flex forwards at the hips until you feel a stretch in the hamstrings.
- At the bottom of the exercise, drive back up to the starting position by extending the hips and driving the feet through the floor.
- Exhale through the most challenging part of the ascent.

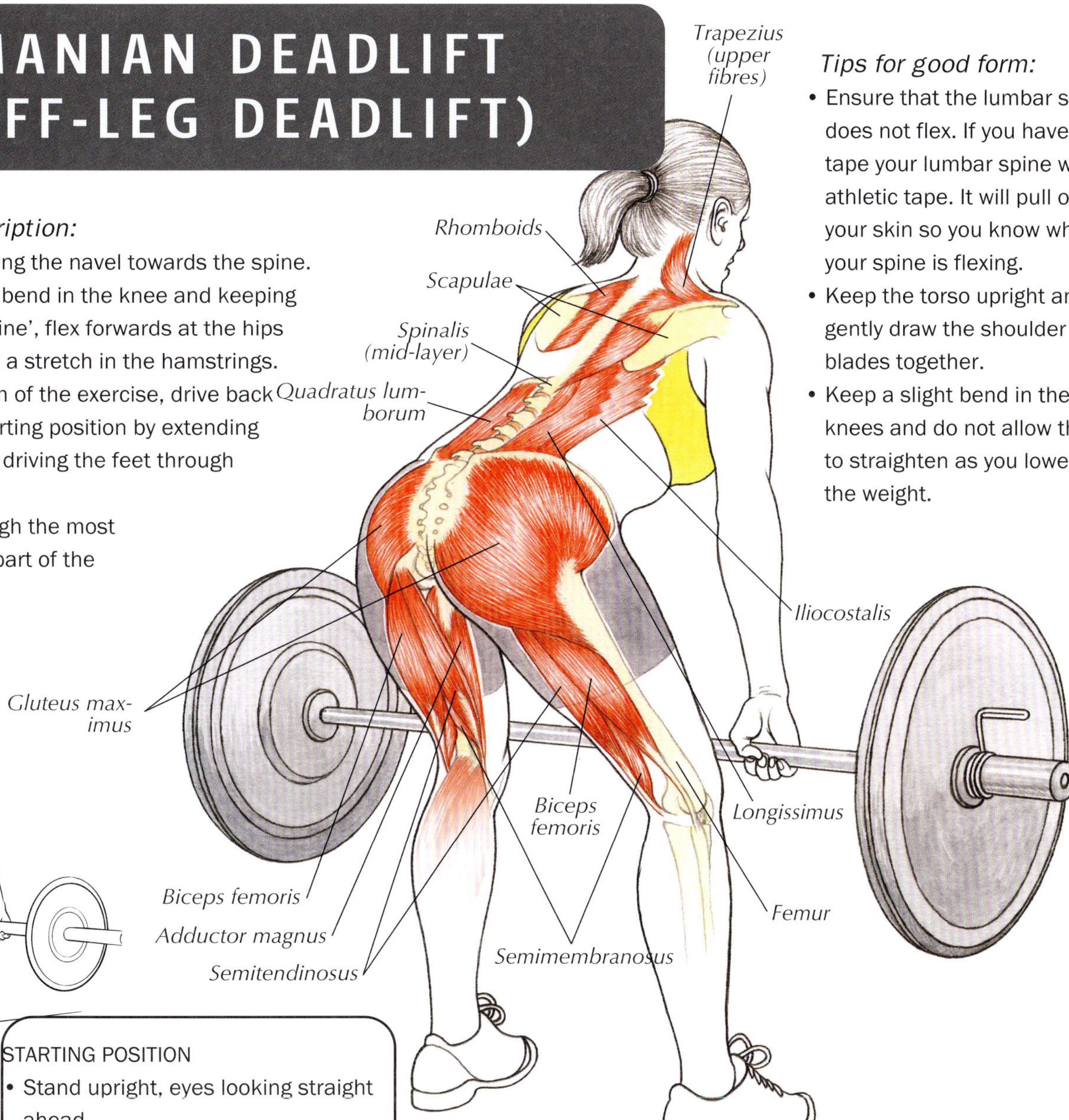

Tips for good form:

- Ensure that the lumbar spine does not flex. If you have to, tape your lumbar spine with athletic tape. It will pull on your skin so you know when your spine is flexing.
- Keep the torso upright and gently draw the shoulder blades together.
- Keep a slight bend in the knees and do not allow then to straighten as you lower the weight.

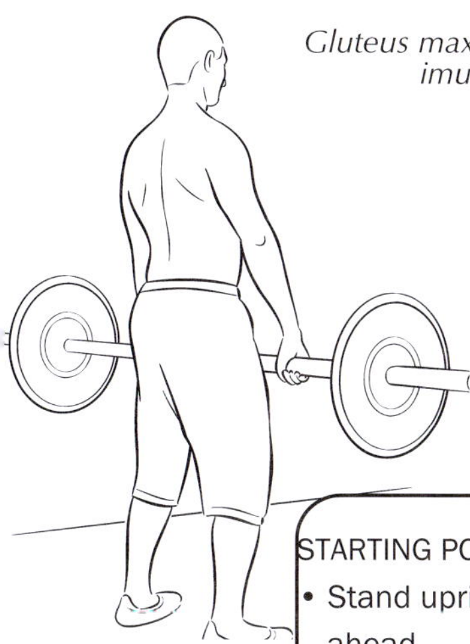

STARTING POSITION

- Stand upright, eyes looking straight ahead.
- Hold a barbell at arms' length (dumbbells can also be used).

ANALYSIS OF MOVEMENT-cialis	*JOINTS*	*JOINT MOVEMENT*	*MOBILIZING MUSCLES*
Joint 1	Hip	Down: flexion, Up: extension	Gluteus maximus, gluteus medius (posterior fibres), biceps femoris, semitendinosus, semimembranosus, adductor magnus (posterior fibres)
Joint 2	Lumbar Spine	Stabilization: extension	Multifidus, spinalis, longissimus, iliocostalis, quadratus lumborum, interspinalis
Joint 3	Scapula	Adduction	Trapezius (middle fibres), rhomboid major and minor
Joint 4	Wrist	Grip: flexion	Flexor carpi radialis, flexor carpi ulnaris, palmaris longus, flexor digitorum superfi

SINGLE ARM CABLE PUSH

Tips for good form:

- Maintain an upright torso, eyes looking straight ahead.
- Keep the forearm in line with the cable and keep the wrist straight.
- Shift your body weight forwards, rotate the torso, then express the push with the arms in one smooth movement.

STARTING POSITION

- Stand facing away from a cable machine, in a low side-lunge position.
- Grab the cable handle with the hand contralateral to the forward leg (for safety reasons grab the handle before you get into the side-lunge position).

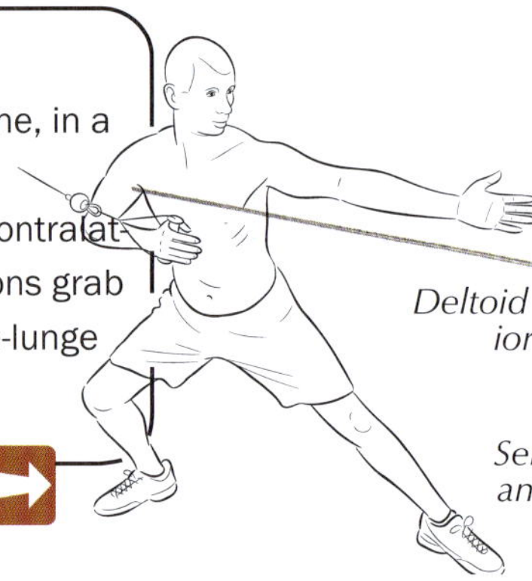

Basic description:

- Inhale, gently draw your navel towards your spine.
- Push off the back foot, driving your body weight away from the machine. Rotate the torso away from the machine and push the cable as if throwing a punch.
  As you push, the opposite arm is driven backwards to create a counter-rotation.
- Exhale through pursed lips as you pass the most challenging part of the push.
- Return the cable to the start position while maintaining the drawing in of the navel and simultaneously inhaling.

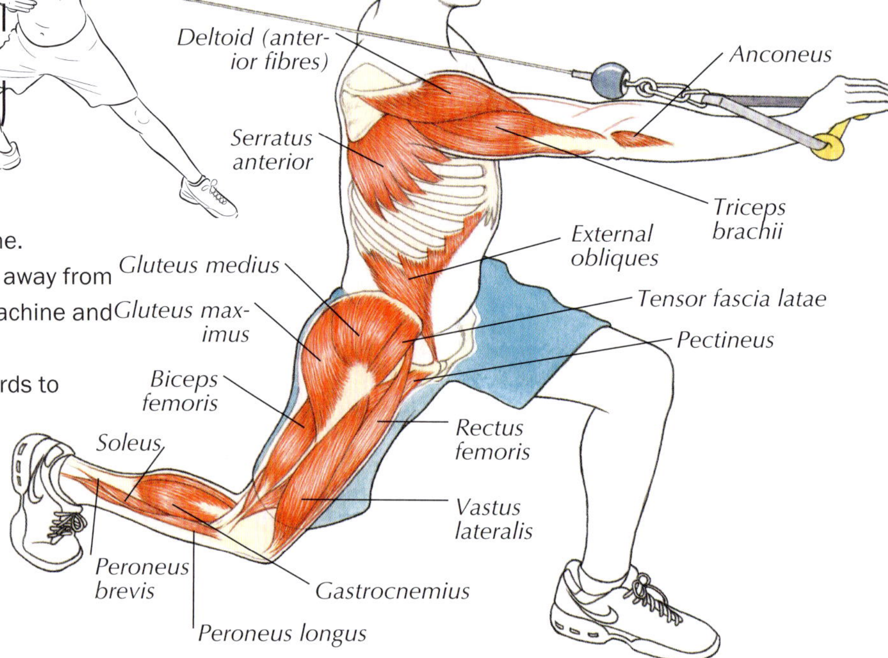

ANALYSIS OF MOVEMENT quadratus	*JOINTS*	*JOINT MOVEMENT*	*MOBILIZING MUSCLES*
Joint 1	Ankle	Back leg: plantarflexion Front leg: dorsiflexion	Back leg: Gastrocnemius, soleus, tibialis posterior, peroneus longus and brevis
Joint 2	Knee	Back leg: extension Front leg: flexion	Back leg: Rectus femoris, vastus medialis, vastus intermedius, vastus lateralis
Joint 3	Hip	Back leg: extension, internal rotation Front leg: flexion, internal rotation	Back leg: Gluteus maximus, gluteus medius (posterior fibres), biceps femoris, semitendinosus, semimembranosus, Gluteus medius (anterior fibres), gluteus minimus, pectineus, adductor brevis, longus and magnus, gracilis, tensor fascia lata
Joint 4	Spine	Rotation	Ipsilateral: Internal oblique Contralateral: Multifidus, rotatores, external oblique
Joint 5	Scapula	Push: abduction Return: adduction	Pectoralis minor, serratus anterior
Joint 6	Shoulder	Push: horizontal adduction Return: horizontal abduction	Deltoid (anterior fibres), pectoralis major (upper fibres)
Joint 7	Elbow	Push: extension Return: flexion	Triceps brachii, anconeus
Joint 8	Forearm	Push: pronation Return: supination	Pronator teres, pronator

SINGLE ARM DUMBBELL SHRUG

Basic description:

- Inhale, gently drawing the navel in towards the spine.
- Shrug the shoulder up on the side of the body holding the dumbbell.
- Exhale through pursed lips as you pass the sticking point.

Tips for good form:

- Keep good torso posture and don't allow the shoulders to round forwards.
- Keep the head still avoiding side-flexion and protrusion of the head.

STARTING POSITION

- Stand up straight with good posture, feet shoulder-width apart, holding a dumbbell in one hand.

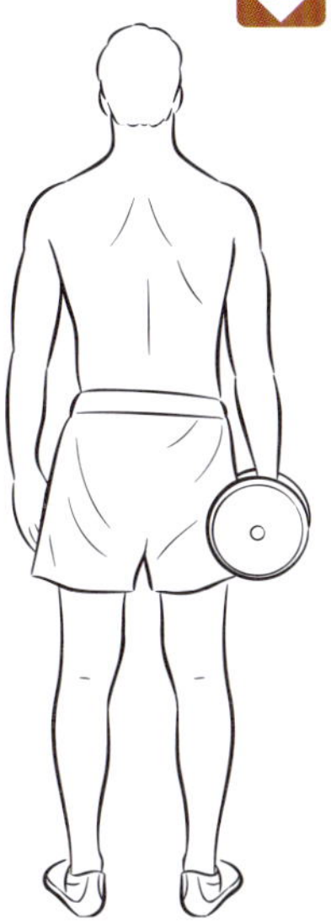

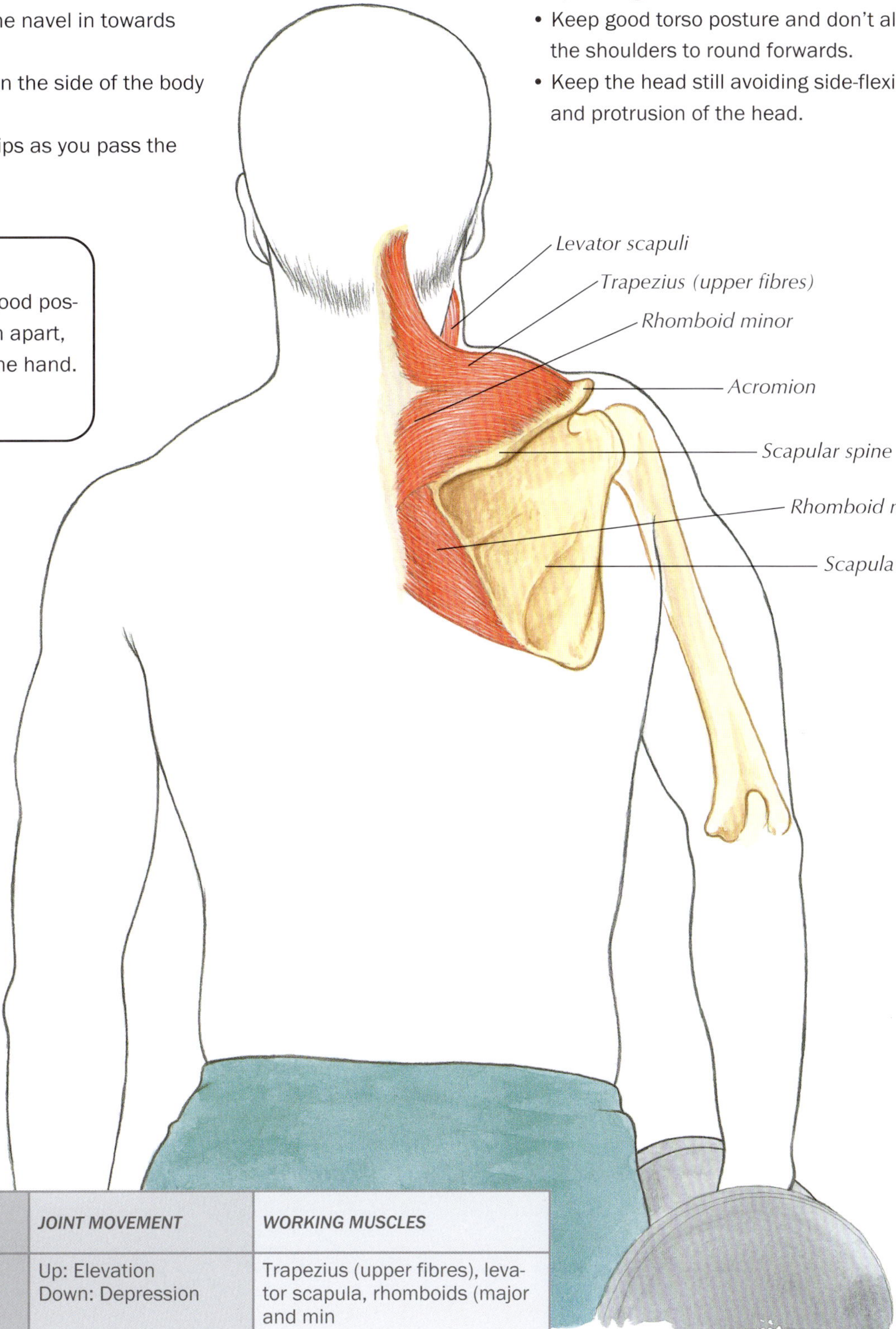

ANALYSIS OF MOVEMENTor)	*JOINTS*	*JOINT MOVEMENT*	*WORKING MUSCLES*
Joint 1	Scapula	Up: Elevation Down: Depression	Trapezius (upper fibres), levator scapula, rhomboids (major and min

SINGLE ARM CABLE PULL

Basic description:

- Inhale, gently drawing your navel towards your spine.
- Push off the front heel, driving your body weight away from the machine, rotate your torso away from the machine and pull the cable as if drawing a bow. As you pull, the opposite arm is driven forwards to create a counter rotation.
- Exhale through pursed lips as you pass the most challenging part of the pull.
- Return the cable to the starting position while simultaneously inhaling and drawing in your navel.

STARTING POSITION

- Stand facing a cable machine, in a low lunge position.
- Grab the cable handle with the hand contralateral to the forward leg.

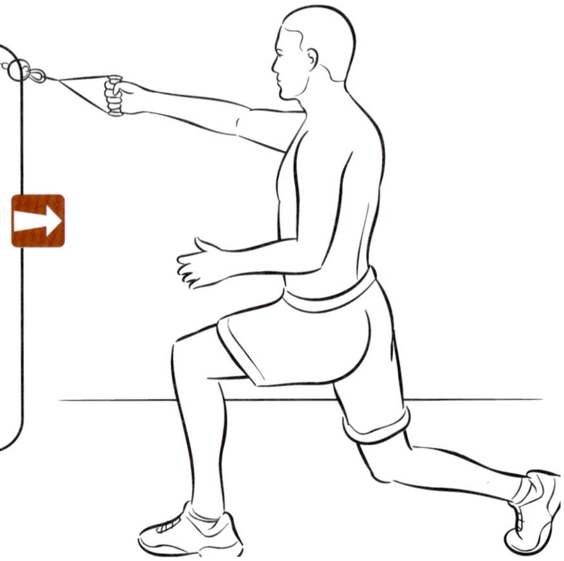

ANALYSIS OF MOVEMENT supinator	*JOINTS*	*JOINT MOVEMENT*	*MOBILIZING MUSCLES*
Joint 1	Ankle	Front: plantarflexion Back: dorsiflexion	Front foot: gastrocnemius, soleus, tibialis posterior, peroneus longus and brevis
Joint 2	Knee	Front: extension	Rectus femoris, vastus medialis, vastus intermedius, vastus lateralis
Joint 3	Hip	Front: extension Back: external rotation	Front: gluteus maximus, gluteus medius (posterior fibres), biceps femoris, semitendonosus, semimembranosus, adductor magnus (posterior fibres) Back: gluteus maximus, gluteus medius (posterior fibres), biceps femoris, sartorius, psoas, iliacus, piriformis, quadratus femoris, gemellus superior and inferior, obturator externus and internus
Joint 4	Spine	Rotation	Ipsilateral: internal oblique Contralateral: multifidus, rotatores, external oblique
Joint 5	Scapula	Pull: adduction Return: abduction	Trapezius (middle fibres), rhomboid major and minor
Joint 6	Shoulder	Pull: horizontal abduction, extension Return: horizontal adduction	Deltoid (posterior fibres), infraspinatus, teres minor, latissimus dorsi, teres major
Joint 7	Elbow	Pull: flexion Return: extension	Biceps brachii, brachialis, brachioradialis, flexor carpi radialis, palmaris
Joint 8	Forearm	Pull: supination Return: pronation	Biceps brachii,

Tips for good form:

- Maintain an upright torso, eyes looking straight ahead.
- Keep the forearm in line with the cable and keep the wrist straight.
- Shift your body weight backwards, rotate your torso, then express the pull with the arms in one smooth motion.

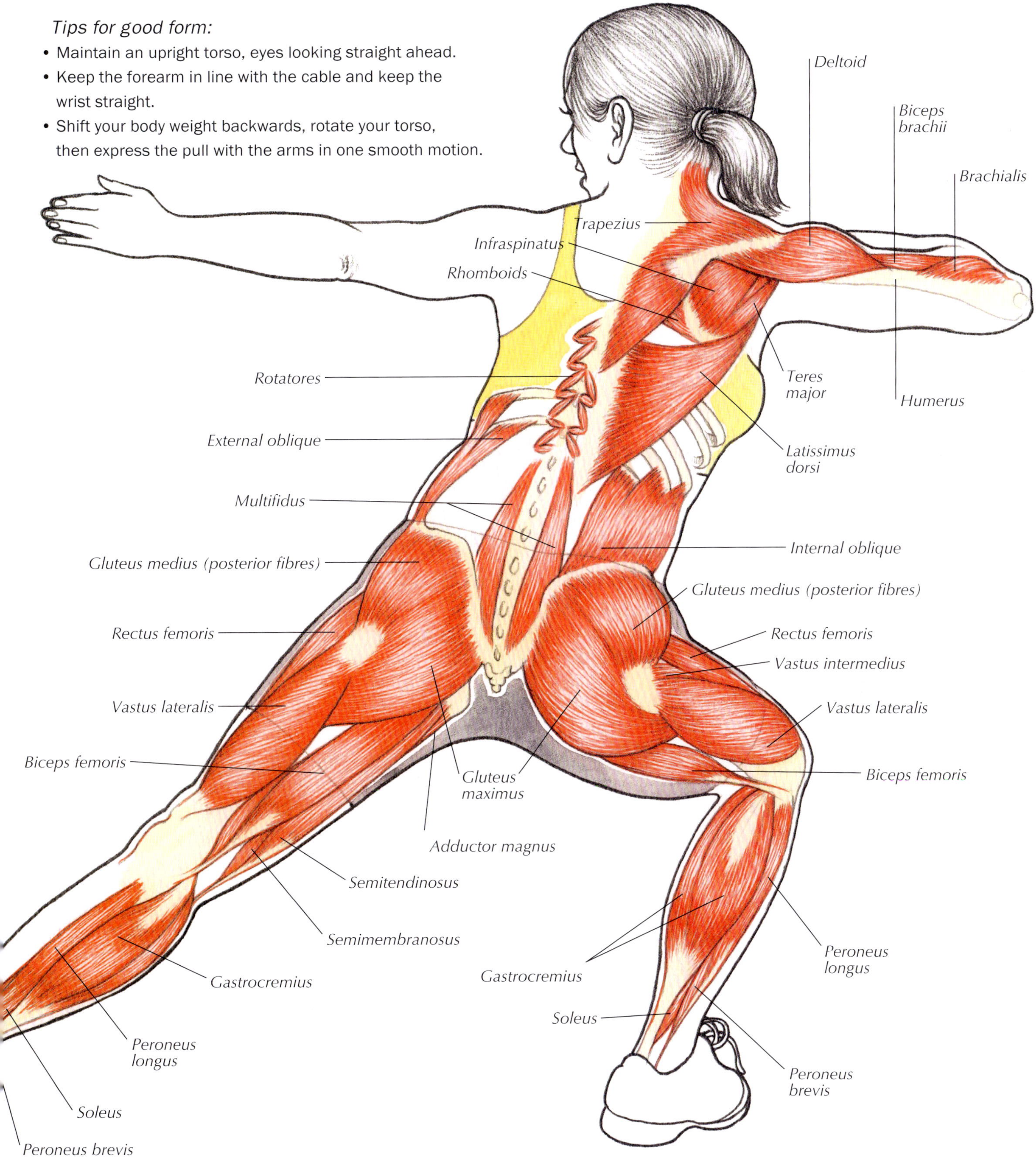

SUPINE HIP EXTENSION ON BALL WITH BELT

STARTING POSITION

- Lie supine with head, neck and shoulders on a Swiss ball, feet flat on the floor, belt around lower thighs.
- Place tongue on roof of the mouth behind the front teeth.

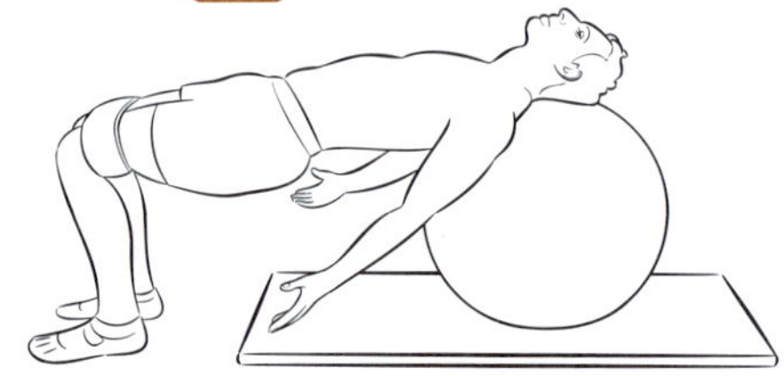

Basic description:

- Inhale, gently drawing the navel in towards the spine.
- Lower the hips towards the floor while exhaling.
- Lower the hips until they are close to the ground. Allow the ball to move slightly.
- Slowly lift the hips back up to the starting position, pushing through the mid-heel of the foot while inhaling.

Tips for good form:

- Keep the shins perpendicular to the ground.
- Drive up from the bottom position by using the gluteals.
- Keep the knees from falling inwards during the movement.

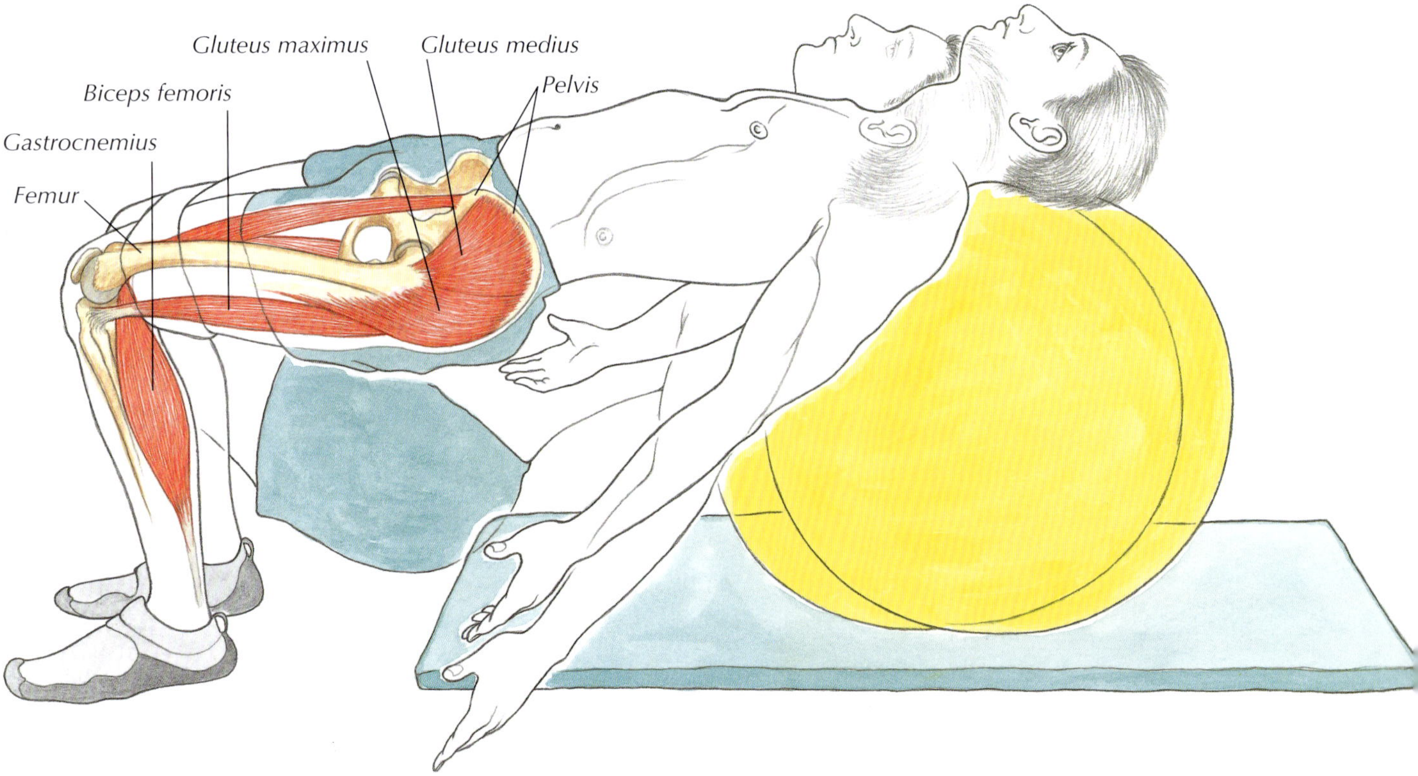

ANALYSIS OF MOVEMENTre-vis	JOINTS	JOINT MOVEMENT	WORKING MUSCLES
Joint 1	Hip	Down: flexion Up: extension	Gluteus maximus, gluteus medius (posterior fibres), biceps femoris, semitendinosus, semimembranosus, adductor magnus (posterior fibres)
Joint 2	Knee	Down: flexion Up: extension	Rectus femoris, vastus medialis, vastus intermedius, vastus lateralis
Joint 3	Ankle	Down: dorsiflexion Up: plantarflexion	Gastrocnemius, soleus, tibialis posterior, peroneus longus and b

WATER JOG-GING

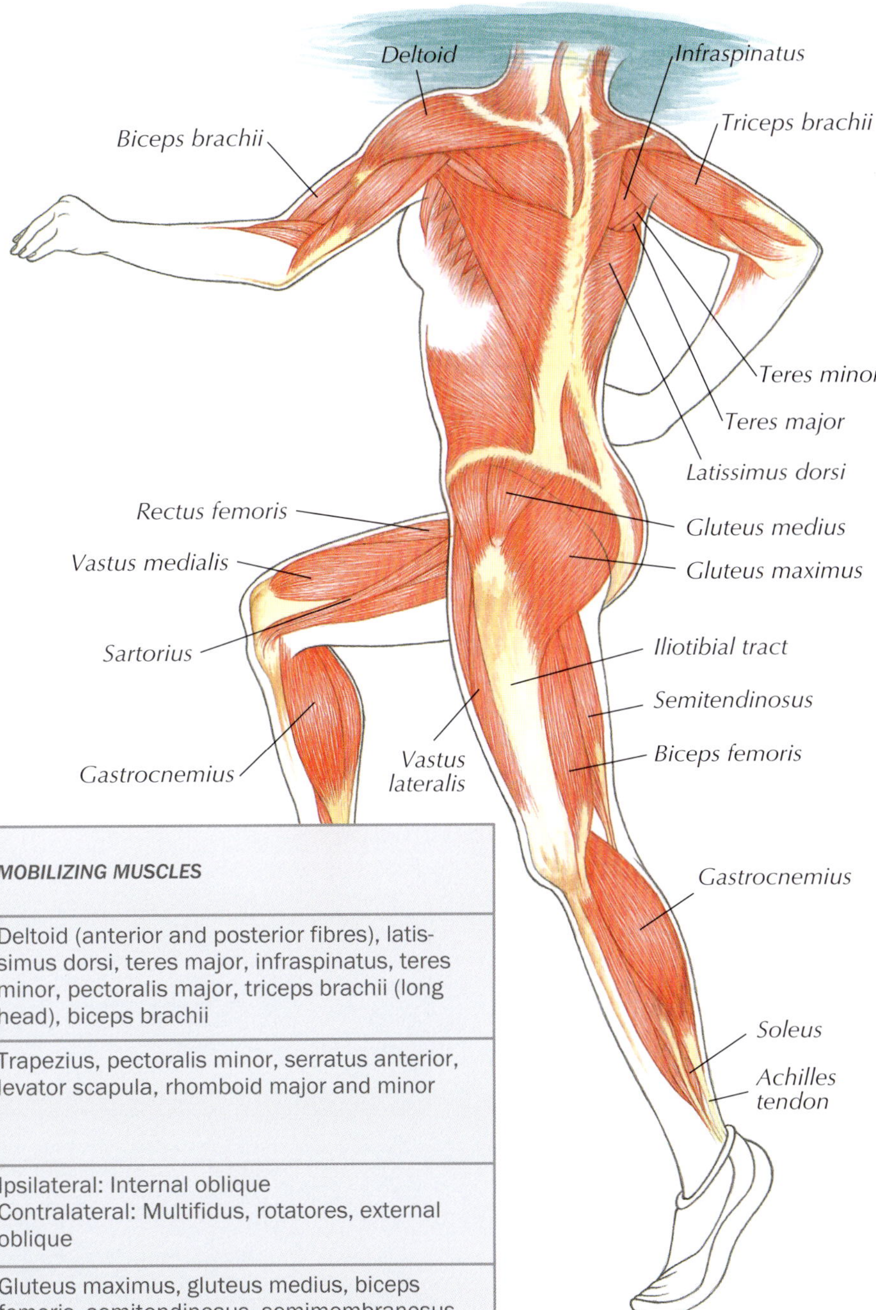

Basic description:

- Begin walking at a comfortable pace that causes you no pain.
- Gradually increase the speed of walking/jogging each session as long as no pain exists.
- You can also use different directions, such as forward, backwards and sideways drills.

Tips for good form:

- Try to use your normal gait pattern as much as possible.
- Keep good joint alignment, especially keeping the knee directly over the second toe.

*ANALYSIS OF MOVEMENT*d brevis	*JOINTS*	*JOINT MOVEMENT*	*MOBILIZING MUSCLES*
Joint 1	Shoulder	Flexion, extension	Deltoid (anterior and posterior fibres), latissimus dorsi, teres major, infraspinatus, teres minor, pectoralis major, triceps brachii (long head), biceps brachii
Joint 2	Scapula	Upward rotation, downward rotation, abduction, adduction	Trapezius, pectoralis minor, serratus anterior, levator scapula, rhomboid major and minor
Joint 3	Spine	Rotation	Ipsilateral: Internal oblique Contralateral: Multifidus, rotatores, external oblique
Joint 4	Hip	Extension, flexion	Gluteus maximus, gluteus medius, biceps femoris, semitendinosus, semimembranosus, psoas, iliacus, rectus femoris, tensor fascia lata, sartorius, adductor brevis, longus and magnus, gluteus minimus
Joint 5	Knee	Extension, flexion	Rectus femoris, vastus medialis, vastus intermedius, vastus lateralis, biceps femoris, semitendinosus, semimembranosus, gracilis, sartorius, gastrocnemius, popliteus, plantaris
Joint 6	Ankle	Plantarflexion, dorsiflexion	Gastrocnemius, soleus, tibialis posterior, peroneus longus and brevis, Gastrocnemius, soleus, tibialis posterior, peroneus longus an

STARTING POSITION

- Stand upright in a swimming pool with the water at waist-height or higher.

WOOD CHOP

Basic description:

- Stand facing away from a cable machine, in a side-lunge position with 70° of your weight on the inside leg.
- Grab the cable handle with the hand furthest from the machine. Place the hand closest on top of the other hand.
- Inhale, gently drawing your navel towards the spine.
- Push off the foot closest to the cable, driving your body weight away from the machine. Rotate the torso away from the machine and twist the cable as if chopping wood.

FINISH POSITION

- Exhale through pursed lips as you pass the most challenging part of the twist.
- Return the cable to the starting position, maintaining the drawing in of the navel and simultaneously inhaling.

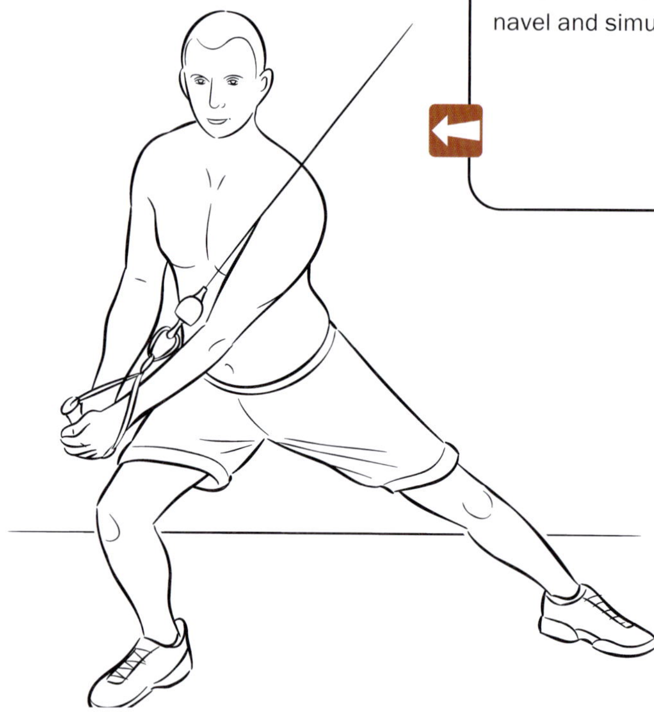

*ANALYSIS OF MOVEMENT*d brevis	*JOINTS*	*JOINT MOVEMENT*	*MOBILIZING MUSCLES*
Joint 1	Spine	Rotation	Ipsilateral: Internal oblique Contralateral: Multifidus, rotatores, external oblique
Joint 2	Scapula	Downward rotation, upward rotation, adduction, abduction, elevation, depression	Trapezius (upper and lower fibres), pectoralis minor, serratus anterior
Joint 3	Shoulder	Extension, flexion	Triceps brachii, anconeus
Joint 4	Hip	Internal rotation, lateral rotation, abduction, adduction	Inside leg: Gluteus maximus, gluteus medius, gluteus minimus, tensor fascia lata, sartorius, pectineus, adductor brevis, longus and magnus, gracilis, tensor fascia lata, semitendinosus, semimembranosus Outside leg: Gluteus maximus, gluteus medius (posterior fibres), biceps femoris, sartorius, psoas, iliacus, piriformis, quadratus femoris, gemellus superior and inferior, obturator externus and internus
Joint 5	Knee	Extension, flexion	Rectus femoris, vastus medialis, vastus intermedius, vastus lateralis
Joint 6	Ankle	Plantarflexion, dorsiflexion	Gastrocnemius, soleus, tibialis posterior, peroneus longus an

Tips for good form:

- Maintain an upright torso, eyes looking straight ahead.
- Maintain a slight bend in the elbows.
- Shift your body weight sideways, rotate the torso, then express the twist with the arms in one smooth movement.

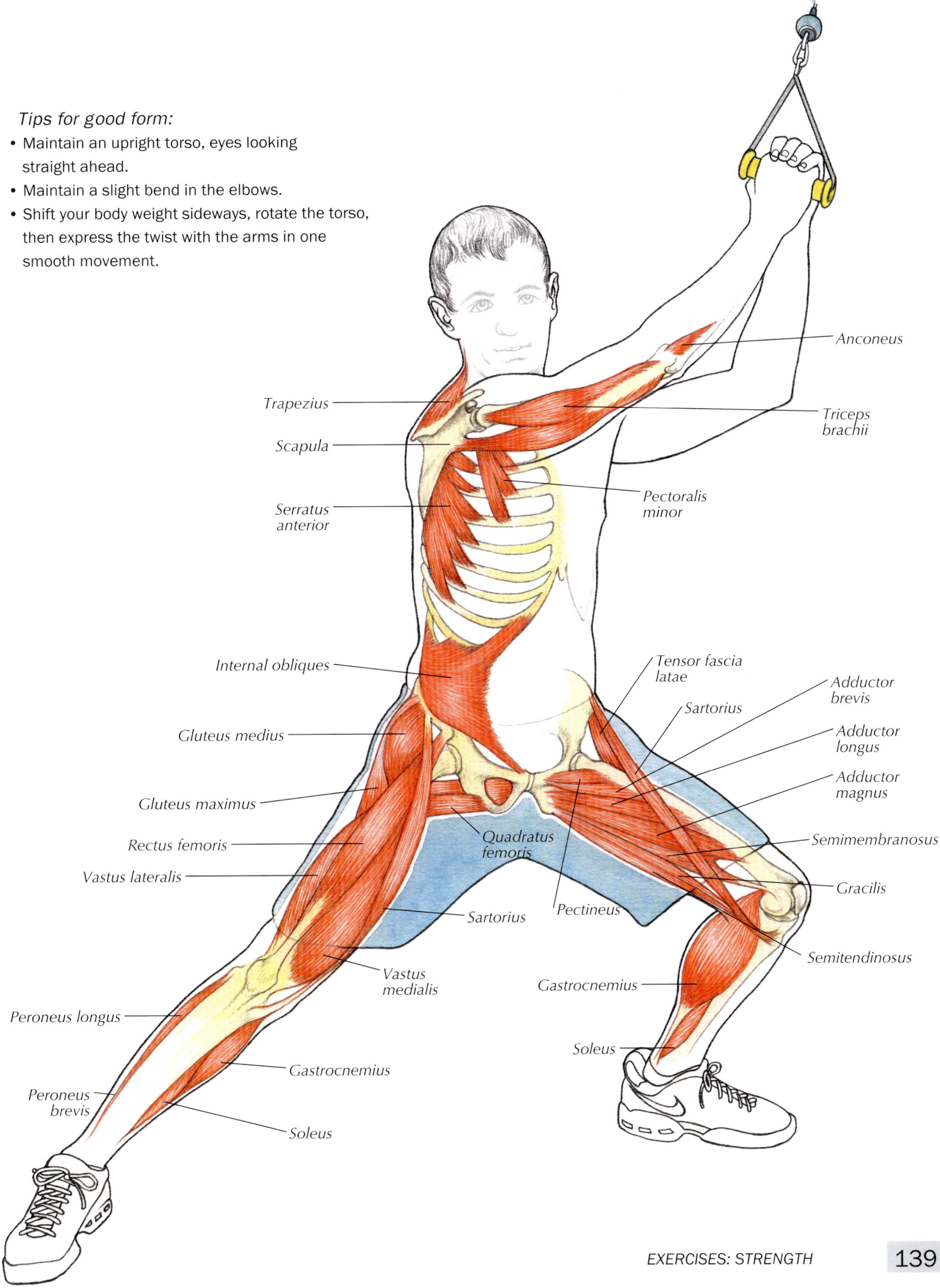

WRIST EXTENSORS

WRIST FLEXORS

Basic description:
- Hold ball with palm facing back.
- Extend the wrist upwards as far as possible without causing pain.
- Slowly lower down into full flexion.

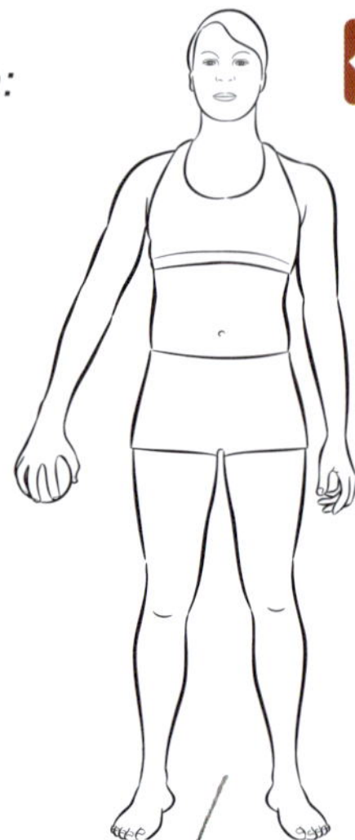

STARTING POSITION
- Stand with feet hip-width apart, holding small medicine ball or dumbbell in one hand.

Tips for good form:
- Keep good torso posture.
- Keep the movements slow and within pain-free ranges.

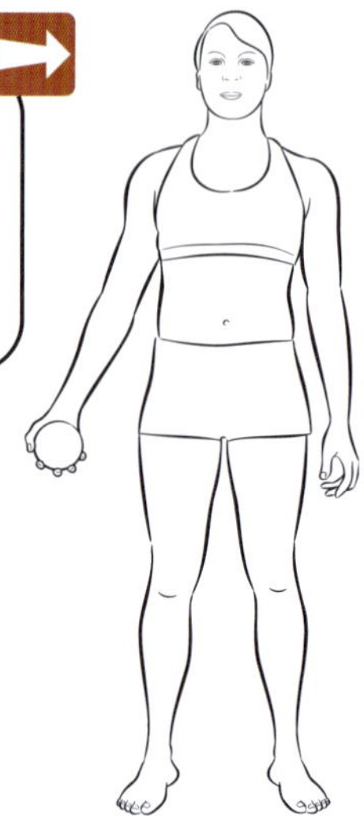

Basic description:
- Hold ball with palm facing front.
- Flex the wrist upwards as far as possible without causing pain
- Slowly lower down into full extension.

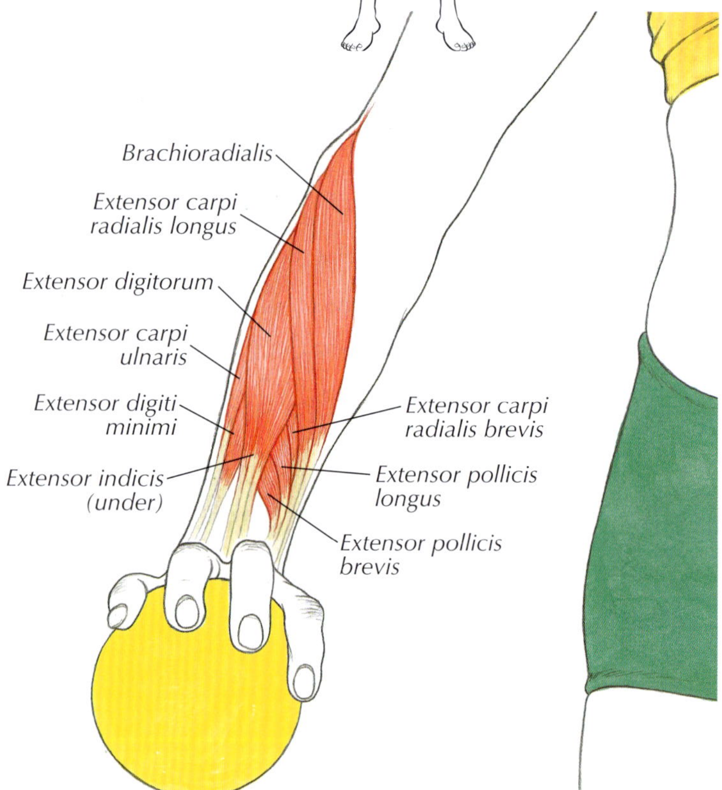

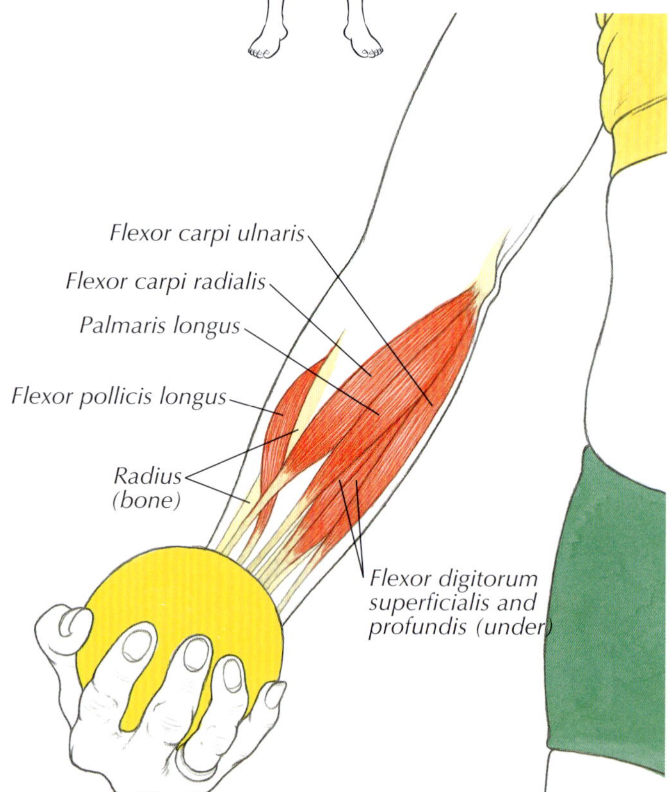

*ANALYSIS OF MOVEMENT*evis	*JOINTS*	*JOINT MOVEMENT*	*WORKING MUSCLES*
Extensors	Wrist	Up: extension Down: flexion	Extensor carpi radialis longus and brevis, extensor carpi ulnaris, extensor digitorum, extensor indicis, extensor digiti minimi, extensor pollicis longus, extensor pollicis br
*Flexors*WristUp: flexion Down: extension Flexor carpi radialis, flexor carpi ulnaris, flexor digitorum superficialis and profundus, palmaris longus, flexor pollicis longus			

GLOSSARY

Compound exercise is a movement that involves a number of joints.

Contralateral refers to the opposite side.

Force closure is the stabilization of a joint created by myofascial (muscle and fascia) action. Often referred to in the stabilization of the sacroiliac joint.

Form closure is the stabilization of a joint created by articular components. Often referred to in the stabilization of the sacroiliac joint.

Gravity pattern (see over-pronation).

Hypertrophy is the increase in tissue size, often referred to as the increase of muscle tissue.

Intensity is a measure of load of an exercise relative to the current level of strength, often measured as a percentage of 1 repetition maximum (1 RM).

Ipsilateral refers to the same side.

Isolation exercise is a movement that involves one joint.

Lower cross syndrome is a postural distortion in the body where the pelvis is anteriorly rotated and the lumbar spine has a hyper-lordosis. The iliopsoas, rectus femoris, tensor fascia lata, sartorius, quadratus lumborum, lumbar erectors are usually short and tight. The lower rectus abdominus, external obliques, gluteus maximus and hamstring muscles are usually long and can be weak.

Metabolic Typing® is way of determining and fine-tuning an individual's optimum diet based on genetic and environmental factors, plus identifying and minimizing potential 'blocking factors' to health.

Muscle spindles are sensory receptors along the length of a muscle, which detect changes in the length of the muscle. Muscle spindles feedback information back to the central nervous system.

Neural drive refers to the number and amplitude of nerve impulses received by a muscle.

Neutral spine is the natural position of the spine when standing without any muscle imbalances, and is achieved when the cervical, thoracic and lumbar spinal curvatures each have an angle of 30–35°.

Over-pronation is a static and/or dynamic posture that occurs when the hip medially rotates, the mid-knee adducts inside the line of the second toe and the ankle pronates significantly from neutral. This is often caused by weakness in the abductors and external rotators of the hip and the abdominal muscles.

Pars articularis is the part of vertebra located between the inferior and superior articular processes of the facet joint.

Passive closure is the stabilization of a joint created by articular components. Often referred to in the stabilization of the sacroiliac joint.

Phasic muscles have a main role in creating movement across joints and in gross stabilization of joints. They have a predominance of fast-twitch muscle fibres, can create high levels of force, are fast to fatigue and tend to lengthen and weaken under faulty loading.

Reflex inhibition is a decrease in reflex activity caused by a sensory stimulus such as pain.

Sensory-motor amnesia is inhibition of muscles caused by long-term lack of stimulus, such as sedentary lifestyle.

Shear force is a parallel stress placed on a joint often in an anterior–posterior or left–right direction. Shear occurs when an applied force produces sliding between two planes. Often referred to in relation to stress placed on the spine.

Swiss ball is an inflated PVC ball used for exercises. It ranges in size: 35–85 cm (14–34 in) in diameter.

Synergistic dominance takes place when a synergist muscle takes over the role of an inhibited prime mover muscle.

Thenar eminence is the group of muscles on the palm of the hand at the base of the thumb.

Tonic muscles' main role is in creating segmental stabilization of the joints. They have a predominance of slow-twitch muscle fibres, create low levels of force, are slow to fatigue and tend to shorten and tighten under faulty loading.

Torsion is a rotational stress applied to an object. Often referred to the rotational force (torque) placed on the spine.

Training volume is the combination of repetitions multiplied by the number of sets and weight (intensity) used over a period of time (workout, week, month).

Upper cross syndrome is a rounded shoulder and forward head posture. The pectoralis minor, sternocleidomastoid, scalene, subscapularis, levator scapula and upper rectus abdominus muscles are usually tight. The rhomboid major and minor, middle trapezius, teres minor and infraspinatus muscles are normally long and may be weak.

Viscera are the internal organs, such as the lungs and liver.

Viscero-somato reflex is a phenomenon where a visceral disorder causes myofascial (muscular) pain.

INDEX

REFERENCES

References

1. Feldenkrais, M., *Body and Mature Behavior*, International Universities Press (1949)
2. Chek, P., *CHEK Golf Biomechanic Certification Manual*, CHEK Institute (1999)
3. Brandon, L. and Jenkins N., *Anatomy of Yoga for Posture and Health*, New Holland Publishers (2010)
4. Balfour, Lady E., *The Living Soil*, Faber and Faber (1943)
5. Lee, D., *The Pelvic Girdle,* Churchill Livingstone (1999)
6. Richardson, C.; Jull, G,; Hodges, P. and Hides, J., *Therapeutic Exercise for Spinal Segmental Stabilization in Low Back Pain*, Churchill Livingstone (1999)
7. Hannah, T. *Somatics*, Perseus Books (1998)
8. Gerwin, R., 'Myofascial and Visceral Pain Syndromes: Visceral-Somatic Pain Representations', *Journal of Musculoskeletal Pain,* Vol. 10, No. 1/2, pp 165–175 (2002)
9. Gracovetsky, S.; *The Spinal Engine*, Springer-Verlag (1998)

Bibliography and further reading

Cash M., *Sport and Remedial Massage Therapy*, Ebury Press (1996)

Chek, P., *The Golf Biomechanics Manual*, CHEK Institute (3rd ed 2010)

Chek, P., (2004) *How, to Eat, Move and Be Healthy!*, CHEK Institute (2004)

Bompa, T., *Periodization – Theory and Methodology of Training*', Human Kinetics (1999)

Chek, P., *Program Design – Choosing Reps, Loads, Tempo and Rest Periods*',CHEK Institute (2nd ed 2011)

Chek, P., *Scientific Back Training– Correspondence Course*, CHEK Institute (2nd ed 2011)

Chek, P., *Scientific Core Conditioning – Correspondence Course*, CHEK Institute (1998)

De Castella R., et al., *Smart Sport – the Ultimate Reference Manual for Sports People*, RWM Publishing Pty Limited (1996)

Ward K., *Hands on Sports Therapy*, Thomson (2004)

www.emedicine.medscape.com

www.eorthopod.com

www.jointpaininfo.com

www.medicinenet.com

www.orthopedics.about.com

www.sportex.net

www.sportsinjuryclinic.net

www.sportsmedicine.about.com

www.wheelessonline.com

www.wikipedia.org

Useful resources

www.bodychek.co.uk The author's website containing articles, newsletters, a blog, online courses, live workshops and resources to aid sports injuries and optimal performance.

www.chekinstitute.com Specialists in advanced education for health and fitness professionals, providing quality information, educational materials and functional training tools.

www.eorthopod.com Detailed articles and videos on orthopedic conditions.
www.orthopedics.about.com Includes a series of detailed articles on orthopedic injuries.
www.sportex.net A professional subscription service giving detailed information and articles on sports medicine and sports injuries.
www.sportsinjuryclinic.net Includes detailed information on many sports injuries and retailer of sports injury products.

Author's acknowledgements

I would like to thank Paul Chek who has been an inspiration, a teacher, a mentor and a great friend. I would also like to thank my parents who have supported me throughout my career. Without their support, I would not be where I am today. I would like to thank Guy and Marilyn at New Holland for their support throughout the project and James, whose artistic talent brings this book to life. I must also thank Juliana Campos, Nicola Jenkins, Paul Read and Rachael Quinlan for modelling for the book.

Please note: the illustrations on pages 30, 34 and 35 are all adapted from original references by Paul Chek and are used with permission.